MW00616911

Yoga exists in the world
because everything is linked.

– Desikashar

Many lovely people have helped me
ensure this book blossoms into reality.
I would like to thank my inspiration,
colleague, teacher, and friend, Susi
Hately Aldous, for not only planting seeds
but also motivating and supporting me
throughout this journey; my chiropractor,
supporter, teacher, and friend, Dr Jeffrey
Scholten, who has been up for anything
and has assisted with the editing,
content, and photos in this book; my
dear friend Roseline Melzer, whose honest
eyes helped develop this book from a
client's point of view; Lorrie Maffey, PT,
who has been an incredible technical
resource and has helped considerably
to make sure this book is thorough and
correct; Jodi Ouellette, whose support,
friendship, and beautiful soul and body
have given this book life and personality;
Susi, Cara, Anne, and Marietta, who
make Functional Synergy such a fantastic
place to be a part of; my wonderful love,
Dennis, and fantastic children, Aidan and
Fiona, who smother me in unconditional
pure love and support and are my "one
true authentic swing." Finally, I would like
to thank my students, who are my real
teachers and inspiration for this book.

– This book is for you all.

Whether you are sitting, standing, walking, or running; moving from one yoga asana to the next; or remaining in one yoga asana for a lengthy period of time, your core stability is enabling you to feel, to express, and to fill out the shape that you are. From the feet to the base of the skull, the muscles that make up your core nestle in to support your spine, your pelvic girdle, and your shoulder girdle; connect your lower ribs to the crests of your pelvis; and connect your arm movements to your leg movements. These muscles provide resilience to your relaxation and softness to your strength. They enable freedom.

That is what this book is about – finding the freedom that comes from gaining deep stability within. Through these pages, Suzette guides you through theory and practice to enable you to develop awareness of where your body is in space without having to look; mobility and strength so your body can calmly and quickly respond to wobbles, turns, and shifts; balance so your body can move from fast to slow and slow to fast with ease and accuracy; and breath so you can find the relaxation within the action, the fluidity within the movement.

It is indeed a physical book, a collection of yoga exercises creating muscular contraction and release. However, as you progress through the exercises you may notice some added benefits – you may find not only that your posture shifts, your breathing becomes easier, your muscles that were once held release, and your muscles that were once weak become strong, you may find that as your body changes, your mind changes as well.

In my years teaching yoga, I have seen it occur many times – with the cultivation of inner stability, new levels of calmness and clarity emerge.

You may have opened this book to relieve issues related to back pain, or to improve your yoga practice as a yoga teacher or student, or you may simply want to become stronger, to become more mobile, and to move around with greater ease. Whatever your situation, you've got a great book in your hands. Suzette is one of the best.

If you have any questions about the exercises, techniques, or theory, or if you want to share your successes, please send an email to our yoga studio, Functional Synergy, at lovelyladies@functionalsynergy.com. We'd love to hear from you.

— **Susi Hately Aldous,** June 26, 2006

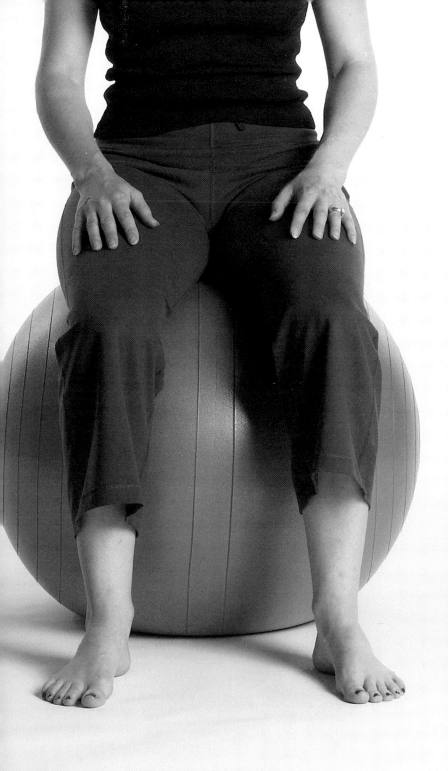

Contents

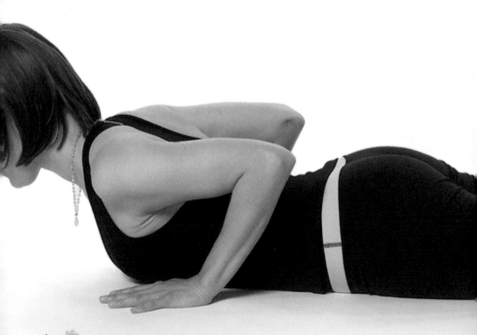

Introduction

We have all heard about the core. It has been the buzzword in the fitness industry for some time now and is permeating all types of physical training and rehabilitation. The core itself is the root of our being, the center of our balance, and in a healthy body, it is also the root of our movements. The core is where we find our intuition, our inner source of knowledge (that "gut feeling"), the center of our souls. In Japanese tradition, the core/belly is referred to as the hara – where the vital energy resides. If you have a good hara, you are considered a centered, balanced individual. Hawaiians call this area the na'au (gut) and believe it connects to your innermost being. In the yoga tradition, this is where we find our root chakra energy and use mula bandha (a pelvic floor–based energy block) during poses to help contain that energy, stabilize it, and draw it up the spine.

This book is designed to teach you about the inner core – how to find it, how to activate it, and how to strengthen and challenge it. You will learn how to draw your root energy through your inner core and stabilize your back from the inside out. You will identify compensating movements and learn how to release and position yourself to allow the ease to flow. You will understand the difference between inner core and outer core and learn how to incorporate both into your training to create a healthy posture and an optimal moving environment. In this way, all your movements will flow safely from the core; your energy will flow freely through your spine and throughout the body. Some of the positive effects you may notice from developing a healthy core include an overall increase in energy levels, a decreased occurrence of injuries, improved posture, diminished muscle tension, and improved performance and quality of life.

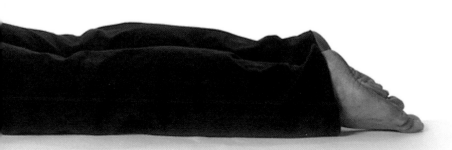

How This Book Is Organized

Yoga for the Core begins by exploring the eight principles of movement endorsed by Functional Synergy. The book is then divided into six chapters. Chapter 1 explains the inner and outer core, how they work, and the muscles involved. Chapter 2 delves into core "helpers," also known as the muscles that tend to compensate when the core is weak or not engaging. Here you'll learn how to release them. Chapters 3, 4, and 5 teach you breathing, releasing, and activating exercises to help you develop and build your core stability. Chapter 6 brings it all together so that you can plan and grow your practice for a strong, supple, and stable core.

Preparing to Practice
Before you begin, change into loose-fitting clothing that is easy to move in. It is best to practice on an empty stomach. Turn off any distractions, including your phone and TV.

What You Will Need
In the beginning stages of this book, all you will need is a space to lie down, a buckled strap or belt, and a pillow. You may need a blanket for under your head. A yoga mat will give you cushioning against laminate or hard floors.

As you progress, a yoga mat will prevent you from slipping. An exercise ball, a BOSU® Balance Trainer, and a long white roller are used to challenge you further by creating a more unstable surface.

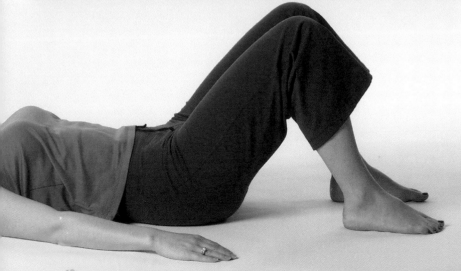

The Eight Principles
of Movement

It is a game that can't be won. Only
played. Play the game. The one only
you was meant to play. The one you
was given when you came into this
world. Now is the time to remember
your swing.

– The Legend of Bagger Vance

The Eight Principles of Movement

At Functional Synergy we follow eight principles of movement to help maintain focus and ease. Based on the natural concepts of anatomy, physiology, and kinesiology, they will help deepen your practice, enhance your exploration, and leverage your body toward greater strength and ease, all while preventing rigidity and injury. As you practice, allow for these principles to be in the back of your mind.

 Principle 1: Nourish Relaxation

Relaxation is the state of mind that brings clarity and focus; it is the state of the body that generates muscle and fascia release, reduces pain, and generates strength. As it relates to creating core stability, relaxation is the key to preventing rigidity, enabling you to let go of unnecessary tension and strain while building supple and resilient stability.

Nourishing relaxation is as simple as becoming aware of your breath. Do this each time you begin your core stability practice. Notice if you are holding your breath, if your breath is shallow, or if it is full and even. However your breath is, practice within its boundaries, knowing that on any given day, it may be different (depending on the day's stresses and activities).

Once you are aware of your breath, the next step is to connect it with your movement. One of the simplest ways to do this is to begin with the spine in mind.

**Principle 2: Initiate Movement:
Begin with the Spine in Mind**

The spine is the fundamental place to begin movement because of its central connection to every piece of the body. At its essence, it is your core.

Each of the spinal vertebrae connects with fascia, blood vessels, muscles, and nerves, which in turn fan in various directions to nourish, stimulate, and balance each part of the body. In a sense, the spine is really a system of skeletal, neurological, electrical, vascular, and chemical input that when balanced and connected creates magically fluid movement, much the same way a well-balanced and connected orchestra creates awe-inspiring music.

As you move, keep this in mind. Think of your spine as your central axis, the hub of your wheel. Allow for your stability to radiate from the spine outward, keeping the image of the orchestra as a backdrop.

This leads us to the next principle, connecting spinal movement with the movement at the largest joints first.

**Principle 3: Connect Spinal Movement with the
Movement at the Largest Joints First**

As you find ease with your breath and awareness, as you feel the spine as the place where your movement will originate from, the next intention is to connect that spinal movement to the shoulder and hip joints. Core stability is often only as good as the mobility we have in our joints, so cultivate pure movement at the shoulders and hips and minimize compensatory actions elsewhere in the body. To help you with this, read on to the next principle.

Principle 4: Move Joints in Their Optimum Range of Motion

All joints have an optimum range of motion. Some move more than others – the shoulder and hip joints move more than the knee or elbow joints; arthritis tends to impede movement. Sometimes one joint will be tight, so others will kick in to compensate. For example, the hip joint may be tight, so to compensate, the lower vertebrae of your spine or the sacroiliac joint may jam or become too mobile.

Honour your body for what it is telling you, and move the joint only in the direction it is intended to move, to the degree it can move today, in this moment. Don't force, remember to breathe easily, and be sure you don't feel pain (see principle 7).

 Principle 5: As You Boost Your Core Stability, Remember to Breathe

Yes, another reminder for you to breathe. If you push too hard in any stage of the exercise the tendency is to hold the breath. If you do, it will have a negative impact on the functioning of the very muscles you are trying to strengthen. In turn, you will become more rigid rather than stable, and you'll cultivate hardness rather than suppleness. As well, your risk for injury will increase. To help prevent this, read on to principle 6.

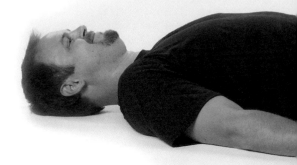

Principle 6: Adopt Relaxed Resilience

Relaxed resilience is akin to effortless effort. It is the opposite of forcing. It requires you to be aware of what is going on in your body while you are moving so that you can make minute changes as you feel you need to. It takes the basic level of relaxation that was cultivated in principle 1, connects it with the spine in principle 2, and facilitates movement at the largest joints first in principle 3, making sure that the movement is optimal as described in principle 4 to help you develop that first level of core stability. As your strength and stability improve, then you'll naturally ramp up to the next level of core stability – with ease and without unnecessary tension.

Relaxed resilience can sometimes be tough to cultivate, particularly if you are a driven individual. If that describes you, the next principle will help you harness your "will" for the good of your body.

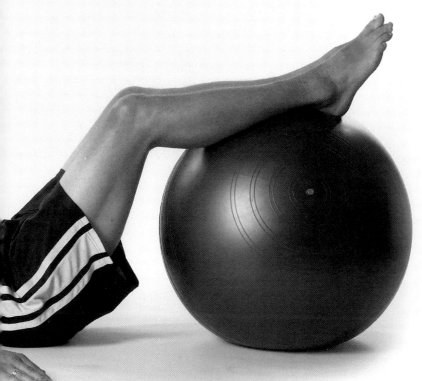

Principle 7: Be Generous with Yourself: Move in Your Pain-Free Range of Motion

Pain is a loaded word with many meanings and interpretations. For the purposes of this book, the aim is for you to distinguish between muscle fatigue (good pain) and searing, tearing, straining, ripping pain (bad pain). This bad pain is the kind of pain that remains for six or seven days following your class or workout and makes you wonder why you signed up. When experiencing pain in this way, mobility and strength will decrease.

To help you settle into your pain-free range of motion, notice the following:

- When you are moving, are you tightening your jaw or neck?
- Is your forehead wrinkling? Or are you trying really hard to keep the forehead from wrinkling (as opposed to gently focusing on the muscles of the core)?
- Is your breath laboured?
- Is there an increase in tension in areas of your body other than the one(s) you are focusing on?

If you answered "yes" to any of these questions, ease out slightly. Although it will initially feel as if you are doing "nothing," you will find greater gains in strength and mobility if you do. Now, we're ready for the final principle. . . .

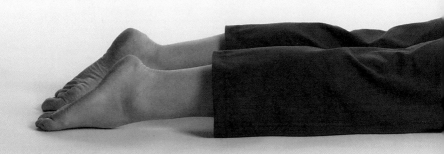

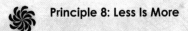

Principle 8: Less Is More

Less is more is not a new concept. Start small, take baby steps, and as you experience success, that success will lead to more success. You will have the momentum to motivate yourself to continue the program. Our experience at Functional Synergy is that this philosophy leads to quicker results.

The preceding was a summary of the eight principles. If you would like to read more detail, please refer to *Anatomy and Asana: Preventing Yoga Injuries,* by Susi Hately Aldous.

Having read through the principles, let's now move into the meat of the theory and practice of stabilizing your core.

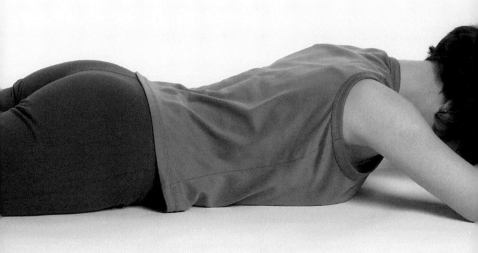

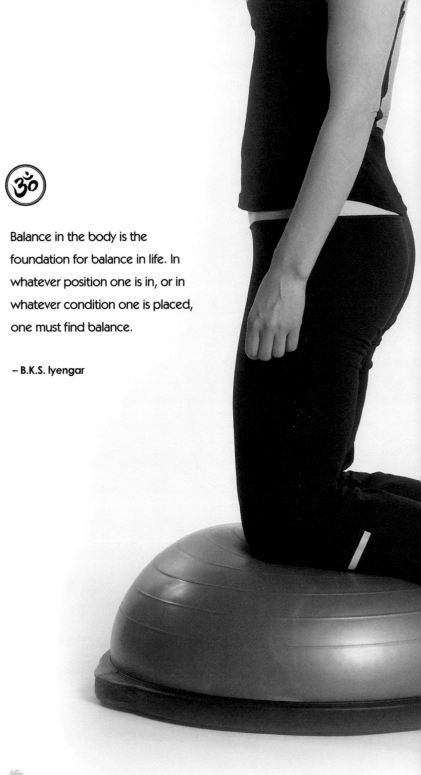

Balance in the body is the foundation for balance in life. In whatever position one is in, or in whatever condition one is placed, one must find balance.

– B.K.S. Iyengar

The Inner and Outer Core

If the basic center which releases
the strength of the whole is missing,
the limbs then have to be con-
sciously directed at will. The effect is
uncoordinated, without inner flow.
There is fatigue and cramp soon
follows.

– Karlfried Graf Durckheim

The Inner and Outer Core

The skeletal muscles in your body perform two different functions: postural and phasic (See chart page 24 and diagrams pages 20-23). The postural muscles are designed for extended use, and they tend toward shortness and tightness. The phasic muscles, designed to move you for short periods of time to complete a task, are predominantly made up of fast-twitch fibers. They tend toward inhibition and weakness and lose their size and strength (atrophy) more quickly than postural muscles. They are also more reactive to injury (Woodruff, 2002).

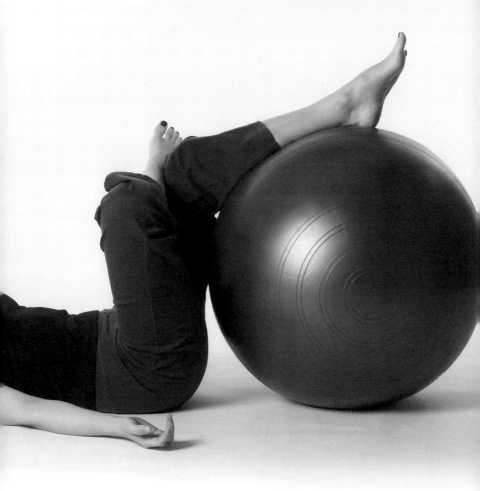

When physical stressors overwhelm your postural muscles, the phasic muscles provide assistance. However, they are not designed for long-term use and can become overworked. When this happens, the phasic muscles become tense, tender, and vulnerable to injury.

The postural muscles are essentially what we refer to as the core muscles. The inner core muscles go one step further, and their predominant function is to stabilize you; they may have other functions such as urinary control (pelvic floor) or breathing (diaphragm), but they do not produce any limb or spinal movements in the body. The outer core muscles create movement in the body (be it limb, shoulder girdle, or spinal movement) as well as a stable and healthy posture. Exercises for these muscles must properly challenge their natural functions and so are very different from traditional strength training exercises. In this book you will learn how to create a strong, stable, aware inner core – with isometric (or static) exercises – and then learn how to develop the outer core around it – with isotonic (or movement) exercises. You will learn how to practice initiating all movements from this stable inner core, allowing you to create stability in an unstable world and respond more optimally to the stresses placed on you in a healthy way.

It is also important to remember that the tendency of postural muscles under stress is to shorten and tighten. This constriction is often a barrier to the development of a strong and stable inner core by limiting your range of motion. It is critical that a complete yoga program focus on both strengthening and lengthening the core muscles to allow you to restore and maintain a natural state of postural balance.

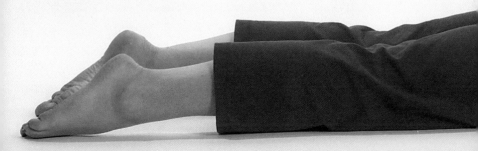

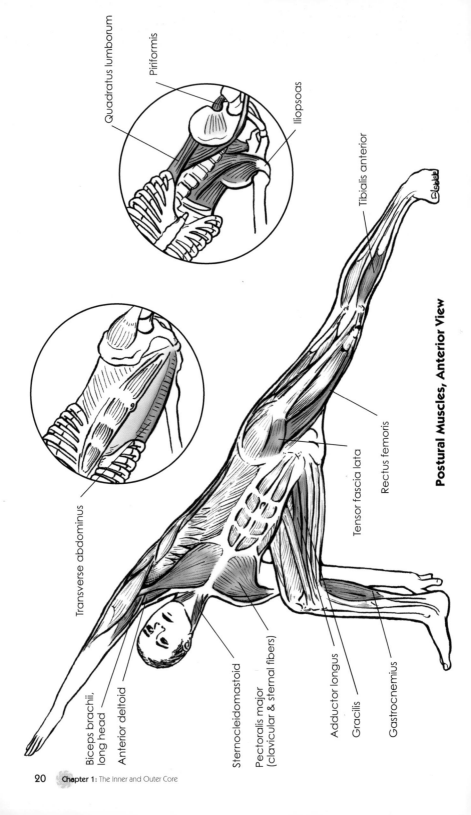

Postural Muscles, Anterior View

Quadratus lumborum

Piriformis

Iliopsoas

Tibialis anterior

Rectus femoris

Tensor fascia lata

Transverse abdominus

Sternocleidomastoid

Pectoralis major (clavicular & sternal fibers)

Biceps brachii, long head

Anterior deltoid

Adductor longus

Gracilis

Gastrocnemius

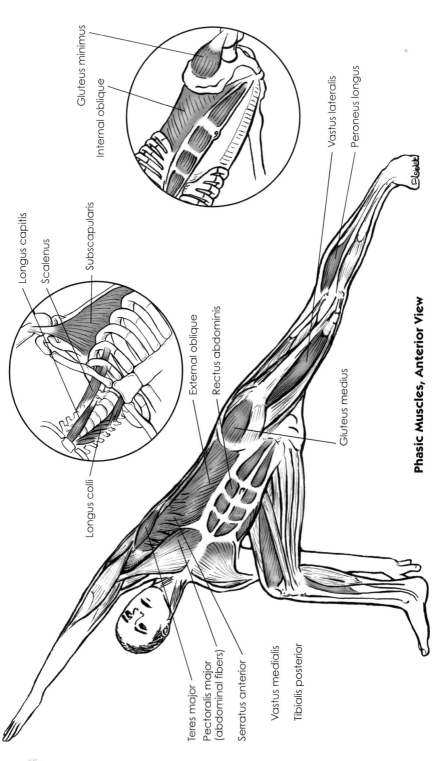

Gluteus minimus

Internal oblique

Longus capitis

Scalenus

Subscapularis

Longus colli

External oblique

Rectus abdominis

Gluteus medius

Vastus lateralis

Peroneus longus

Teres major

Pectoralis major
(abdominal fibers)

Serratus anterior

Vastus medialis

Tibialis posterior

Phasic Muscles, Anterior View

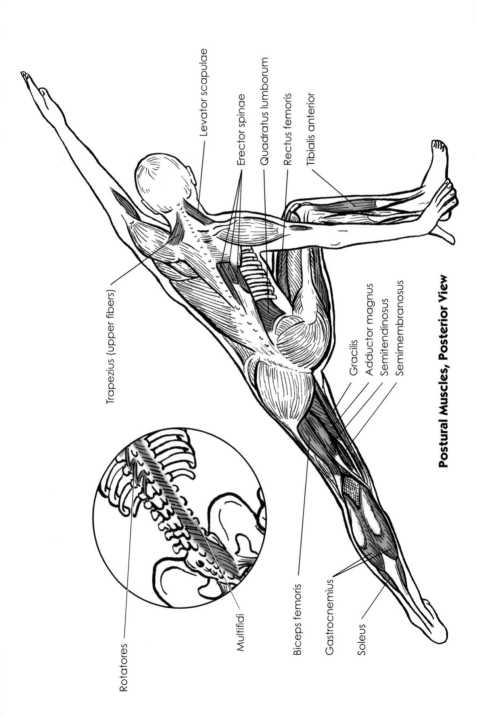

Levator scapulae

Erector spinae

Quadratus lumborum

Rectus femoris

Tibialis anterior

Trapezius (upper fibers)

Gracilis

Adductor magnus

Semitendinosus

Semimembranosus

Postural Muscles, Posterior View

Rotatores

Multifidi

Biceps femoris

Gastrocnemius

Soleus

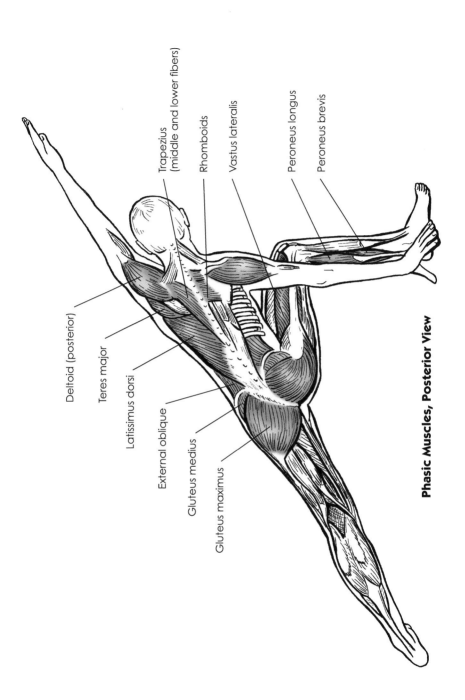

Deltoid (posterior)

Teres major

Latissimus dorsi

External oblique

Gluteus medius

Gluteus maximus

Trapezius (middle and lower fibers)

Rhomboids

Vastus lateralis

Peroneus longus

Peroneus brevis

Phasic Muscles, Posterior View

(Janda, 1983; augmented by Lorrie Maffey, 2006)

Muscles with Mainly POSTURAL Function	Muscles with Mainly PHASIC Function
• Sternocleidomastoid • Upper fibers of trapezius • Levator scapulae • Flexors of the upper extremity: pectoralis major (clavicular and sternal fibers), anterior deltoid, long head of biceps • Quadratus lumborum, erector spinae group, rotatores, multifidi • Transversus abdominis • Hip flexors: iliopsoas, rectus femoris, tensor fascia lata • Piriformis • Hip adductors (one-joint muscles only) • Hip extensors: all three hamstring muscles • Plantar flexors: gastrocnemius, soleus • Tibialis anterior	• Longus colli and capitis • Scalene muscles (vary from postural to phasic) • Pectoralis major (abdominal fibers) • Extensors of the upper extremity: posterior deltoid, teres major, latissimus dorsi • Middle and lower fibers of trapezius • Subscapularis • Rhomboid • Serratus anterior • Abdominals: rectus abdominis, internal and external oblique • Gluteus maximus, medius, minimus • Vastus medialis and lateralis • Tibialis posterior • Peroneus group (fibular)

Keep in mind that although scientists classify muscles into two groups, our aim in increasing inner core stability is to identify the source of muscle response in addition to the response itself.

The Inner Core

The inner core is made up of the diaphragm, anterior pelvic floor, transversus abdominis, and multifidi muscles. There is still some debate as to whether other muscles help make up the inner core as well, but for this book we will limit the discussion to the functions of these muscles, upon which most researchers and health practitioners agree (Richardson et al., 2004).

The inner core muscles help create a stable pelvis and a stable spine, and they can reduce potentially traumatic rotational movements. They are also critical for ensuring that the intra-abdominal contents do not leak or become herniated. Many people refer to this stability as the "powerhouse" of the body. The area is of critical importance because when it is not working properly, other muscles attempt to compensate. Since these muscles are not designed to contract and relax this way, they do so ineffectively, which can lead to further compensation and inactivation of the inner core. This has been shown to possibly result in chronic low back pain; hip and knee injuries; shoulder and neck tension; and repetitive strain injuries (RSI) in the shoulder, neck, or arm due to posture and compensation changes. Following are some of the reasons people develop inner core dysfunction:

1. Just one episode of debilitating low back pain.
2. Gastrointestinal tract infection caused by long- or even medium-term gluten intolerance has been shown to inhibit the abdominal wall. Other gastrointestinal tract irritations caused by digestive system parasitic or fungal infection, food allergies, food additives, or genetically modified foods can also produce the same effect.
3. Stress incontinence.
4. Premenstrual syndrome and childbirth.
5. Deconditioning or the use of nonfunctional fixed-axis exercise equipment in an improper manner (weight-stack exercise machines found in almost all fitness facilities – e.g., leg press or chest press).

As you can see from this far-from-exhaustive list (Wallden, 2004), revisiting education and activation of the inner core should be incorporated into everyone's lifestyles.

Becoming Aware

Looking at the components of the inner core individually, let's investigate your awareness of each.

The Diaphragm

When you breathe from the diaphragm, it contracts on the inhale and relaxes on the exhale. Located at the bottom of the ribs, the diaphragm attaches to the low back by two pillars (or crura) on the bodies of the lumbar vertebrae (L1–L4). When you inhale, the diaphragm flattens out and opens up the bottom of the lungs; this causes a vacuum effect, and the air rushes in through the nose and mouth to fill up this new space. It also causes the abdominal contents to be pushed out of the way, and as a result you feel the belly rise.

The diaphragm – considered a primary respiratory muscle that can work continuously without fatigue – is assisted by the intercostals (muscles between the ribs and the abdominal muscles). This is why our abdominals and ribs can be sore after a hard run, a good laughing session, or a bad cough. Our secondary respiratory muscles include the thin scalenus anterior in the neck, the pectoralis in the chest, the sternocleidomastoid (from the mastoid just behind the ear to the top of the sternum), and the upper trapezius, which runs from the base of the skull to the top of the shoulder blades. These muscles are smaller and more delicate than the primary respiratory muscles. The secondary muscles can act powerfully when needed, but they tire quickly and easily. If they try to become the primary muscles, it can result in tension (chronic and acute), decreased lung volume, a feeling of instability, and a change in posture (Farhi, 1996).

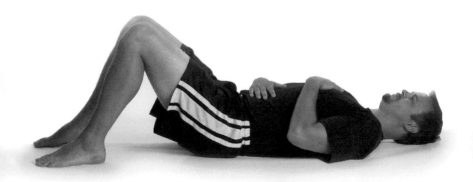

Inquiry: Lying on your back, place one hand on your chest and the other on your belly. *Can you feel the belly move? Which hand moves first, and which hand moves the most?* By focusing on the belly, you can transfer the work from the upper body to the diaphragm.

Notice how this feels in your body and the emotional response you get from breathing from your diaphragm and then from your secondary respiratory muscles. Try this while standing up to see if you can also notice a change in your stability and ability to feel grounded.

Another way to feel the diaphragm and the belly breath is to lie on your tummy in crocodile position, with the legs extended behind you. Cross your arms in front of you so your bottom ribs contact the floor but the rest of your ribs extend upward. Rest your head on your forearms. See if you can feel the breath in the belly. *Can you also feel the spot where the diaphragm attaches to your back?* In this position, your intercostal muscles, your abdominals, and most of your secondary respiratory muscles are already extended, so it is much harder for them to contract to assist in breathing. You are forced to breathe from your diaphragm.

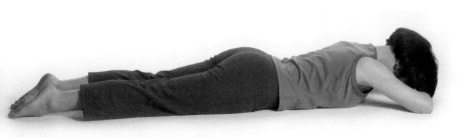

The Yoga Breath vs. the Pilates Breath

For many people who have experienced yoga and Pilates, the difference in breath patterns can be confusing. By understanding why each breath is how it is, you can learn to use the breath to assist yoga poses and Pilates exercises with the greatest awareness and effectiveness. I am trained in hatha yoga and STOTT PILATES®, so I will speak from my training.

The breath pattern in Pilates and yoga acts to release any unnecessary tension in the body. You want to avoid breathing shallowly into the upper portion of the rib cage. Breathing low into the abdominal cavity can cause the abdominal muscles to completely relax, thereby making them unable to protect and stabilize the back during the exercise.

Anatomically, during exhalation the rib cage closes in and down while the spine flexes slightly. Thus we encourage the exhale on spinal flexion during yoga and Pilates. During inhalation the rib cage opens up and out while the spine extends, and so we encourage an inhale on extension. Sometimes we will reverse this in Pilates to maintain abdominal recruitment and support the lumbar spine.

In Pilates we breathe three dimensionally into the lower rib cage (back and side ribs) to allow us to create awareness and initial activation and then increase the abdominal involvement in the movement as the diaphragm assists in the abdominal connection. This may take the form of initiating the pelvic floor and the abdominals on the inhale and moving on the exhale. As we become more aware and increase our abdominal strength, we eventually reverse the breath to increase the challenge to the abdominals. Think of it as a gradual progression to stability. We can also move on the exhale to start and then speed up the movement once the pattern has been established, moving on the inhale as well.

In yoga, the breath is used for energy transformation. Pranayama focuses entirely on this idea. As it relates to core stability, we want to encourage the pelvic floor to contract as the rib cage expands with each contraction of the diaphragm, thereby creating stability as well as drawing up root energy. We may also create a pelvic floor lock (mula bandha) throughout a pose or series of poses to create endurance and strength. Both are incredibly useful breathing techniques that can lead to a strong, stable core.

The Pelvic Floor and Pelvic Diaphragm

Many people have lost their awareness of or their ability to control the pelvic floor. You need the pelvic floor muscles to contract so you can bend from the hip instead of the sacroiliac joint, stabilize the pelvis during movements, initiate your inner core, and improve bladder and rectum control. These are the muscles you would activate if you were taking a midstream urine sample (holding longer than 3 seconds). You need to be able to activate and close all pelvic floor sphincters (i.e., close the openings). The muscles sling around the openings to create support for the perineal body, which can be damaged by childbirth or surgery. If you think of it as a support for the bladder, uterus, and bowels, you can understand that a strong yet tension-free pelvic floor can prevent prolapses and loss of bladder and bowel control. You may have function and be pain free, but without a sense of what is happening you may develop problems during menopause or experience sacroiliac pain.

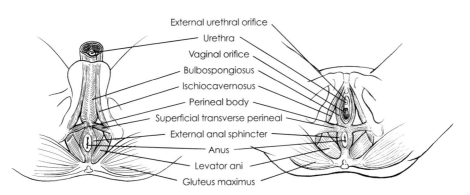

External urethral orifice
Urethra
Vaginal orifice
Bulbospongiosus
Ischiocavernosus
Perineal body
Superficial transverse perineal
External anal sphincter
Anus
Levator ani
Gluteus maximus

Inquiry: To feel the anterior pelvic floor, start by lying on the floor on your back with your knees bent. For women, on an exhale draw up the front half of your pelvic floor, known as the anterior pelvic floor. Men need to "draw the crown jewels up toward the center of the body." Both men and women can think about pulling away from an ice cube just in front of the pubis bones. Try to relax the buttocks. Feel this lift through the center of the body as if you are drawing the energy and contraction up through the middle of you. (See *Anatomy and Asana: Preventing Yoga Injuries* by Susi Hately Aldous for more information on the anatomy of the pelvic floor and the pelvic diaphragm.)

Wait 10 seconds between contractions – you want to ensure complete relaxation before contracting again. If you find you are able to contract only once, you may not be relaxing completely and may be retaining tension in your pelvic floor. Try contracting the anterior pelvic floor, and then try to contract just the posterior pelvic floor (anus). Note if you have an increased awareness and/or activation in the front or the back. The posterior pelvic floor muscles are the most vascular, and since these muscles wrap around the anterior pelvic floor muscles, contracting the back can help you contract the front. It may help to think about pulling forward from back to front (or drawing an imaginary tail through your legs and up your body).

Try contracting the pelvic floor muscles in different positions (legs wide, legs crossed, lying on your tummy, sitting on a chair, standing). A change in position may create the resting length necessary to let you contract those muscles. A physical feeling against the pelvic floor can also help – try sitting on a fitness ball or BOSU® Balance Trainer.

Once you have increased your awareness and activation, develop your ability to contract over time (endurance without losing intensity), your speed (number of squeezes), and your strength (level 10, level 5, and level 3). Ensure you come down to resting level between contractions. (Taken from the Exercising Your Pelvic Floor Workshop, as taught by Meaghan Evans, BScPT, 2006.)

Once you have established a connection and awareness of your pelvic floor, lie on your back and notice the connection between the diaphragm and the pelvic floor.

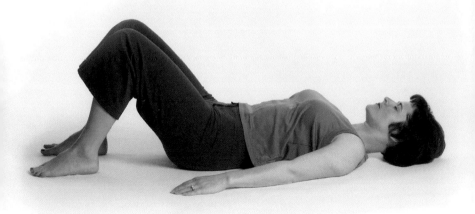

Can you feel the breath through the pelvic floor or a movement with the breath? Be aware of the pelvic alignment. *Is the pelvis level? (That is, are the pubis bones level with the front hip bones?) Can you feel a connection between the pelvic floor and the eyes? The neck?* This is what we also refer to as the pelvic diaphragm, and it is this low level of contraction without other compensations (eye or neck tension, change in pelvic alignment, or change in diaphragm contraction) that we are eventually looking for when we activate our inner cores (a level 2 or 3 out of 10).

Transversus Abdominis

The transversus abdominis covers the front of the abdominal wall from the pelvis to the bottom ribs. It runs across the body from the iliac crest and bottom ribs to the other side. When this muscle contracts, you sense a continuation of the drawing up feeling you got with the pelvic floor. In fact, you need to activate the pelvic floor to properly contract the transversus abdominis muscle.

Inquiry: Drawing up *Activating* Place your fingertips on your anterior iliac crests (front hip bones). Move your fingers just to the inside of the bones (toward the belly button). When the anterior pelvic floor and then the transverse abdominal muscles contract, you may feel an upward contraction or movement under the fingertips on the anterior iliac crests. Feel the contraction from the base of the pelvis to the bottom of the ribs. There should be no change in the position of the spine or pelvis (do not tuck, or posteriorly tilt, the pelvis) – just the stability created from the inner core.

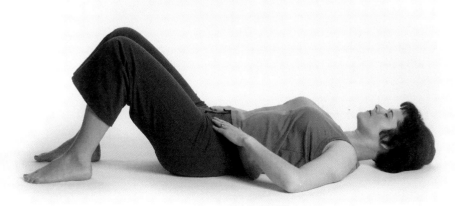

Multifidi Muscles

The multifidi muscles run up the spine and cover 1 to 5 vertebrae at a time (Bogduk, 1997). They stabilize the spine, helping to control localized intersegmental spinal movement. Picture them as a woven ladder running up the spine, all the way from the sacrum to the axis (C2).

Inquiry: To contract these muscles, you need to intensify the drawing up feeling at the spine. Lie on your side, placing one hand on your tummy and the other on your low back just above the pelvis. See if you can draw up and through the low back without moving the pelvis or spine and pushing your back into your hand. You can also feel the contraction in your back as you intensify the contraction in your transversus abdominis.

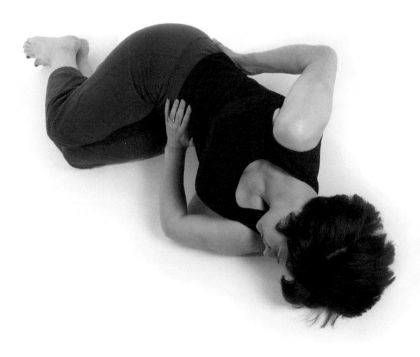

Also, in a standing position, stand on one leg with the other leg lifted 5 to 10 inches out to the side. Place one hand on your low back at the top of the pelvis (the other hand can rest on a support or be on your lower belly to feel your core activate on the front as well). Rotate your lifted leg five times in both directions. Do this with your core relaxed and again with your core activated. *Can you keep your low back from moving against the rotational movement of the leg?*

Variations: Practice inner core activation while lying flat on your back, then try it lying on your tummy, seated, and standing (single-leg and double-leg stance).

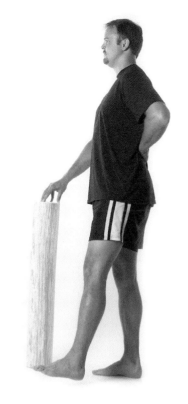

You need to be able to create this stability in all movements; *are there certain positions that are easier or harder for you?*

Summary: Putting It All Together – Stabilizing through the Inner Core
You now have created stability from the bottom (pelvic floor), top (diaphragm), front wrapping around to the sides (transversus abdominis), and back (multifidi). You may have noticed that in a well-functioning spine and muscular system, all the described muscles are recruited with any of the described movements. All these muscles work in harmony to provide stability for the torso and therefore the body.

Now as you practice these activation movements, watch for other movements as well. *Can you keep your neck and shoulder area relaxed? Do your feet, forehead, or legs tense up?* Keep practicing releasing the other areas and isolating the inner core. These other compensatory movements can give us clues as to bad habits we have learned. Because bad habits result in chronic conditions, start by reteaching the body the basics before moving on. It will not take long for the body to relearn the proper pathways (most people notice a change in minutes and a significant change in a week).

Inner Core Strengthening and Awareness Poses

The following exercises will bring together the concepts in this chapter.

Marching Abdominals *Activating*
Marching abdominals is one of the best exercises to increase strength and awareness in the inner core. It is the exercise that all my clients begin with, regardless of their fitness level. It can be very humbling but also very effective.

Start by lying on your back, with your knees bent and feet flat on the floor. Place your fingertips on the front pelvic crest (anterior superior iliac spine – ASIS) on either side. Bring your fingers 1 inch toward the belly button, just inside of the ASIS.

Draw up the inner core, and feel this under your fingertips. Lift one foot off the ground approximately 1 to 4 inches (just take its weight off the floor), and see if you can maintain a stable, nonrocking pelvis (this is another example of the multifidi stabilizing the pelvis against rotational movement). Lower the leg to the ground and repeat on the other side. Keep changing legs, ensuring there is no rocking or dropping of the pelvis when you lift or lower the foot.

To increase the challenge, lift the hips 2 to 4 inches off the floor into Little Bridge Pose (Setu Bandha Sarvangasana). Try lifting alternating feet, keeping the spine and pelvis stable.

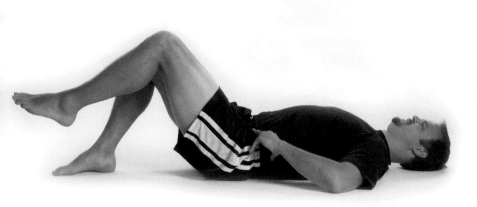

Hip and Knee Release *Activating*

The hip and knee release also helps you feel the stability of the pelvis against limb movement. Lying on your back as for marching abdominals, pretend there is a glass of red wine resting on your pelvis (and you are wearing white!). Drop one knee 4 to 6 inches out to the side without spilling the wine. Repeat a few times before switching to the other side.

Can you keep the pelvis stable and the neck tension free? Does the other leg move to counterbalance the moving leg? Try to isolate the stability in the pelvis and keep the rest of the body still and relaxed. If this is difficult, just think how challenging walking with a stable pelvis is for your body.

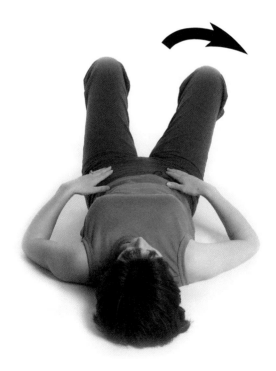

Table Pose *Activating*

By activating the core in the Table position, you can feel how the transversus abdominis muscle must contract and pull the abdominal contents up and in. You are working against gravity in this position and will feel the motion differently, thereby changing or increasing the challenge.

Start by placing the knees under the hips and the hands under the shoulders so you are in the Table position with a neutral spine. On the exhale, without changing the alignment of the spine, draw up from the pelvic floor to the bottom of the ribs *(fig. 1)*. Feel how the abdominal contents come into the body. Inhale and let it all go – just relax the belly once again without changing the spinal alignment *(fig. 2)*.

This is an incredible exercise for pregnant women. It not only develops support for the growing uterus but also helps prevent diastasis recti and low back pain.

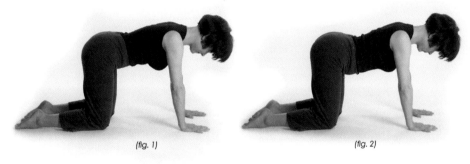

(fig. 1)   (fig. 2)

There are two ways to activate the inner core: abdominal bracing and abdominal hollowing. Abdominal bracing is used when you brace the low back to lift something heavy. It is a pulling in toward the spine of the transversus abdominis muscles. Bracing is incredibly useful for squatting but would be counterproductive for gait-based activities because it limits your mobility. Abdominal hollowing refers to activating the inner core in its entirety – it is how we use the inner core throughout this book. Whether to brace or hollow is a less critical question than the fact that you should contract and stabilize the inner core before you move. People who contract the inner core after the outer core (or not at all) are at risk for decreased performance and increased injury.

Releasing the Outer Core "Helpers"

The trick is to find your swing.
Now somewhere in the harmony
of all that is – all that was – is all
that will be.

– The Legend of Bagger Vance

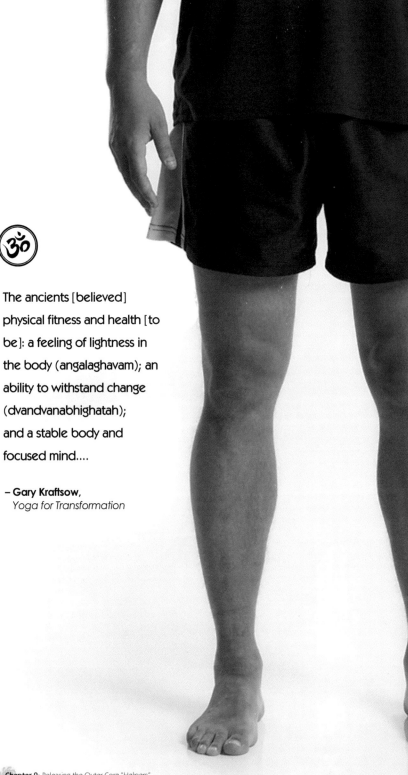

The ancients [believed] physical fitness and health [to be]: a feeling of lightness in the body (angalaghavam); an ability to withstand change (dvandvanabhighatah); and a stable body and focused mind....

– **Gary Kraftsow,**
  Yoga for Transformation

Releasing the Outer Core "Helpers"

If you have been improperly utilizing the inner core through either dysfunction or lack of activation or strength, other muscles in your body start to activate to help out. These could be secondary breathing muscles, as listed in the previous chapter, or muscles surrounding the hips to stabilize the pelvis and low back, for example. The body is incredibly effective at learning how to compensate. Unfortunately, these long-term compensations can lead to destabilization, changes in alignment, chronic tension, and pain. As you are learning how to activate the core, make sure you do not activate other muscles or strengthen a dysfunctional activation. We will look at two of the most common areas that like to assist; however, keep in mind that there may be others to work with in your body. It is important to recognize and feel the body as a whole and actively look for compensations in each pose and movement. We can then learn to deactivate compensations.

Pelvic Girdle Area

The hip flexors (iliopsoas, rectus femoris) like to activate as you stabilize the pelvis during hip abduction (moving the leg away from the midline of the body) and hip adduction (moving the leg toward the midline of the body). To ensure the activation you are producing is from the inner core and is in fact "pure," it is important that the hip flexors relearn how to stay relaxed during movements. If they do activate, they can pull on the pelvis and low back and rotate the pelvis, moving it out of alignment. For most people, one direction is easier than the other. Use one of these movements (the one you can do easily) to learn how to feel pelvic stabilization and thigh movement without the hip flexors activating; use the other (the one you find challenging) to relearn how to release the hip flexors. This is the way you are supposed to move – you just need to learn how to flick the switch and turn the compensating muscles off. As you develop your core strength and practice on a regular basis, you will find that these moves become easy, and you will return to natural movements. It is also a good idea to come back to these exercises every so often to see if you have returned to bad habits as you increase your intensity in other exercises and as you develop natural movement strength.

Try the three exercises on the following pages to see if your hip flexors can remain relaxed.

Exercise #1: Pressing into a Strap *Activating*
(or a Belt or Tie from a Housecoat) – Hip Abduction

Lie on your back with your knees bent, feet in line with buttocks. Place a strap around your mid-thighs and tighten just so the legs can relax into the strap. With your hands on the crease between the top of your thighs and pelvis, lift one leg 1 inch off the ground. You should feel your hip flexors contract and bulge out (this is their natural movement). Return the foot to the floor and feel the muscles relax. Repeat with the other leg. Position your fingertips right on the hip flexors to feel them if they start to activate.

Keeping the hip flexors relaxed, press into the strap. Press subtly at first and then a little more. Press until you feel your hip flexors activate or your pelvis start to move. Do not try to relax while activating, just start again and don't go as deep. You will (or eventually will) be able to feel your inner core stabilize your pelvis, your buttocks activate into the strap, and your hip flexors remain still. Try this exercise with your legs wider, legs closer, knees apart, feet together. Eventually move on to your side to work against gravity (see the clam exercise).

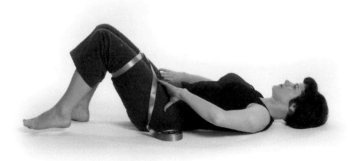

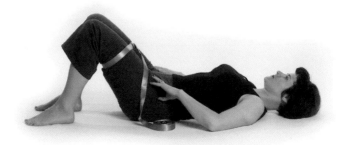

Exercise #2: Pressing into a Pillow *Activating*

With your body in the same starting position (on your back, knees bent, feet in line with buttocks), remove the strap and place a pillow between the knees and hips. Be sure the pillow is firm and is not touching the knees. Find the hip flexors again, and this time press into the pillow. You will (or eventually will) be able to feel your inner core stabilize your pelvis, your inner thighs activate into the pillow, and your hip flexors remain still. Try this exercise with different sized pillows.

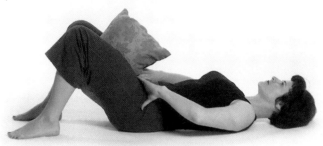

Exercise #3: The Clam

Once you are able to keep the hip flexor muscles relaxed during hip abduction while lying on your back, try working against gravity through the clam.

Lie on your side with your hips and shoulders stacked, neck supported. Knees and hips are bent to 90 degrees. Place your top hand on your hip flexor; notice if there is activation in your hip flexor in this starting position (you may need to place a pillow or prop between your legs until you can find the position where your hip flexors relax). Keeping your feet together, activate the external rotators of the hip (gluteus maximus) and lift the knee off the other leg. Make sure the hip flexors stay relaxed (completely, not just a little – remember this is a subtle movement, and more is not better). Find the range of motion that you can work with, and then gradually increase it as you learn how to keep that switch flicked off.

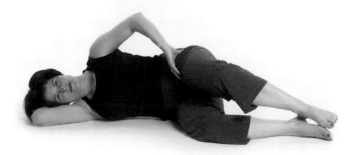

Neck and Shoulder Girdle Area

The shoulder girdle and neck are connected through the spine and musculature of the torso. You need them to work together, but you also need them to learn how to work independently. It is very common to feel the shoulder girdle tense up as you are activating the pelvic girdle. There are some things you can do to release these muscles before and during your practice. This will lead to being able to release them during the rest of your day and life.

Try the following three exercises to help release the neck and shoulder girdle area.

Exercise #1: Supporting the Head While Lying on Your Back
Release

When lying on your back, it is important to maintain a neutral alignment in the cervical spine (neck). The alignment you are striving for is for the top of the lip to be in line with your forehead, with the chin slightly below your forehead. You can also get someone to check that the inside of the ear is in line with the center of your shoulder.

You need this position to be relaxing rather than straining. To release the neck muscles and allow the muscles to start to move into alignment, try lengthening from the back of the head (where the neck and head come together), softening your neck with your breath, or adding a prop. You can place a blanket under your head to bring the ears in line with the center of your shoulders or raise the head and shoulders off the ground by folding the blanket in two levels. You need to make sure that the cervical spine holds its alignment with the thoracic spine and that you have not propped up the head too high, leading to a new kind of neck tension. A small roll under the neck also helps relax the neck and hold it in alignment. If you are using a prop, make sure you also use your breath to release the neck muscles into position.

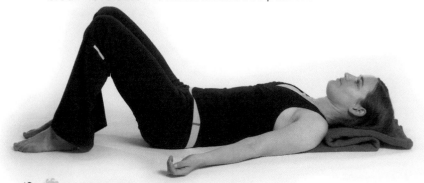

Exercise #2: Diaphragmatic Breathing

By bringing your breath into the belly, you can relax and release the secondary breathing muscles. The following are examples of diaphragm breathing exercises:

- Belly breathing – chapter 1, page 26
- Crocodile breathing – chapter 1, page 27
- Table breathing on ball – chapter 4, page 63

Exercise #3: Neck and Shoulder Releasing Exercises

Try some of the neck and shoulder releasing exercises in this book after your breathing poses to further release these muscles.

- Neck and shoulder release – chapter 4, page 61
- Cat with ball – chapter 4, page 63
- Eagle on ball – chapter 4, page 69

Increased Total Body Awareness

Releasing the outer core will enhance your total body awareness and will help activate your inner core. Try the following as you practice: Breathe softness as you focus on your body. *How are your toes, the palms of your hands, your forehead, and the corners of your eyes?* There are many areas in the body that we tend to tighten or change alignment of when we have our awareness in other areas. Try noticing the connection between one area in the body and the way the rest of the body reacts.

Have you ever noticed how your nose gets itchy when you are carrying something heavy with both hands?

Gather your strength in one point only – in the lower belly.

– Master Okada

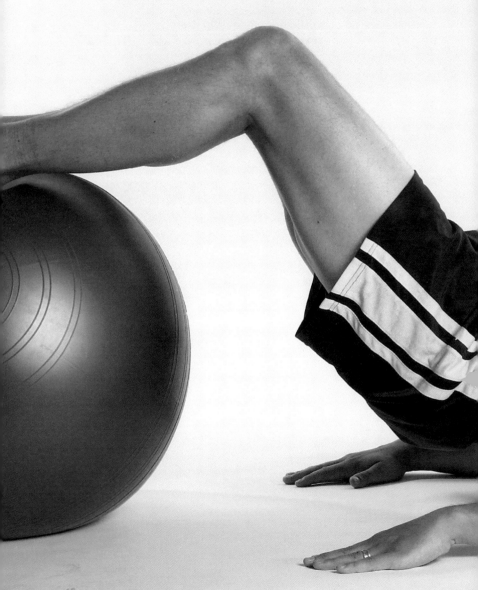

Building Stability

Be soft in your practice. Think of
the method as a fine silvery stream,
not a raging waterfall. Follow the
stream, have faith in its course. It
will go its own way, meandering
here, trickling there. It will find the
grooves, the cracks, the crevices.
Just follow it. Never let it out of your
sight. It will take you.

– Sheng-yen

Building Stability

When you train your core, you create a stable base inside the body from which all movement can then begin. This stable base will allow your muscles to react properly, thereby increasing your ability to avoid injury in moments of instability. Life is full of these unstable moments: taking a step, slipping on ice, picking up a piece of paper, or sneezing while looking off to the side. To best train your body to deal with an unstable and constantly changing environment, you need to train it the way you use it. This is called the SAID training principle (specific adaptations to imposed demands), and it is common to exercise programs (to become a better rower, you need to row).

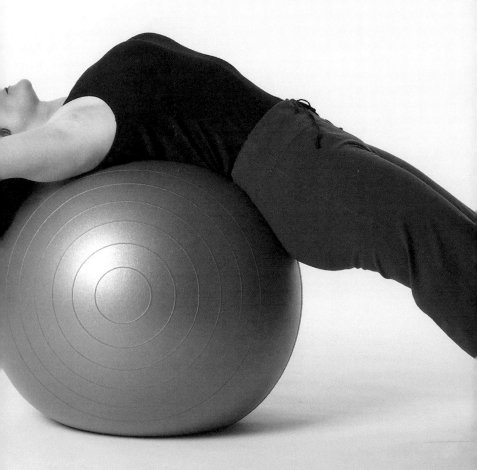

Once you have created the awareness of where your inner core is and how to activate it, you then need to learn how to do this in the circumstances you find yourself in on a regular basis. This is where stability training comes in. By placing yourself in a position of instability, you will increase the activation of these muscles and thus the training response. In other words – you will get better results that are applicable to life.

When practicing and learning how to create stability, it is important to understand how to alter the difficulty level of individual exercises. The following points demonstrate how to increase the challenge posed by any exercise (Lorrie Maffey, 2006). Keep them in mind as you work with each of the poses in this book.

- Decrease your base of support (e.g., one-leg stance, feet closer together, hands by your sides instead of outstretched).
- Decrease the stability of the surface you are working on (e.g., stand on a pillow, soft blanket, mattress, or balance board, or add more air to your ball).
- Increase the length of levers (e.g., extend your arms over your head, or move from a bent leg to a straight leg when lying on your back).
- Increase the resistance you are working with (e.g., hold a weight in your hand or strapped onto the ankle).
- Increase the speed of movement while maintaining proper position.
- Increase the complexity of the movement (your mind is occupied with more things at the same time).
- React to an external stimulus (e.g., someone tossing you a ball while you perform the pose).

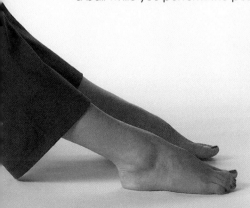

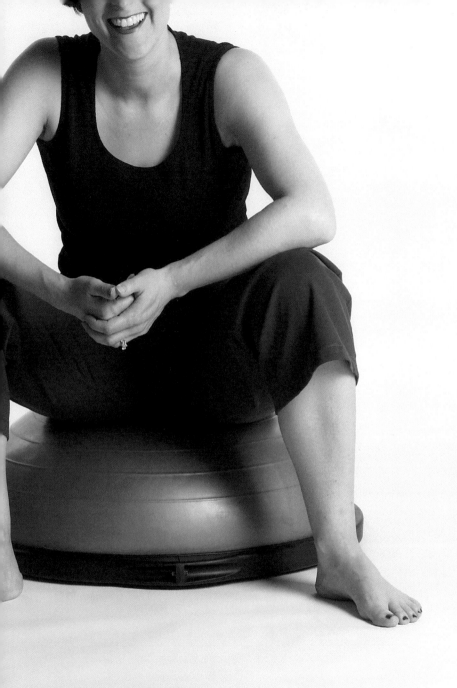

Mountain Pose (Tadasana) *Activating*

Begin by standing, balancing your weight evenly over the foot –
from the ball of the foot to the heel – with both feet on the ground.
Bend your knees and hips, keeping your knees forward and in line
with the second toes (as if you are going to sit on a chair). As you
straighten your legs, draw up your inner core as you push your legs
into the ground. Repeat this until you feel equal balance of weight
in your feet (front to back, inside to outside, left to right), the
activation in your inner core, and the strength in your legs. Try to
breathe easily and softly, holding the activation in the inner core or
reconnecting it with each exhale.

Be aware of how grounded you are, how stable you have become,
how easy your posture feels. Try the pose with and without the
involvement of your inner core, and feel the difference. *Can you
push your legs into the ground without activating your inner core?
Can you activate your inner core without pushing your legs into the
ground?*

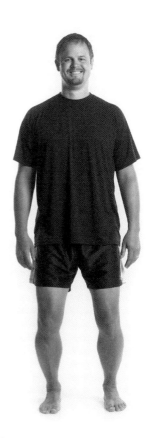 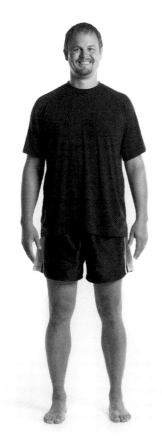

Tree Pose (Vrksasana) *Activating*

This balance pose incorporates a rotational component at the hip, thereby making it a little more challenging.

From Mountain Pose, transfer the weight to the right leg. Be sure not to lose the height in the hip and waist, and keep your core active. Lift your left leg so only your toes are touching the ground, thinking tall through the right side of the body. Without moving your pelvis or spine, rotate the left knee out and place your hands in front of your heart in namaskar (prayer position). Slide the foot up the inner thigh while you lift your left knee as high as possible without losing the pelvic or spinal alignment.

Incorrect   Correct

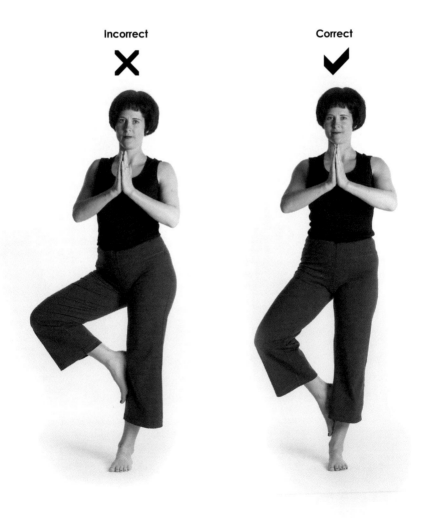

Now extend both arms above your head to the sky in a wide alignment, or stay in namaskar.

Focus your mind on lifting out of the right hip, constantly drawing up the inner core on the exhale and softening the shoulders out of the ears. Stay here for 4 to 12 breaths, then repeat on the opposite side.

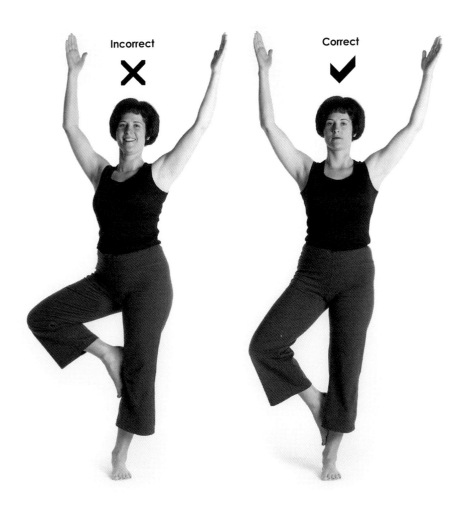

Warrior III Pose (Virabhadrasana III) *Activating*

Warrior III is another balance pose that incorporates an increased challenge for the core and low back as you try to maintain pelvic stability in a forward folding position.

From Mountain Pose, transfer your weight to the right leg without losing the height in the hip and waist, keeping your core active. Place the toes of your left leg on the ground, lifting your left heel up, thinking tall through the right side of the body. Flex the left hip slightly so the leg is lifted in front of you just off the floor. Reach both arms above your head to the sky, feeling the length in the body but also the space between the ears and the shoulders (keep the shoulders down and open).

Fold forward from your right hip (not the low back). Your left leg will swing back and lift up off the ground behind you, and your arms will stay in the same alignment with your head as in the beginning position. Make sure you do not rotate (open) the hips upward. Focus on your inner core and pelvic alignment to keep the hips level. Keep tall through the right hip; you should feel as if you are bringing the left hip down. Hold this position for 4 to 12 breaths, then repeat on the other side.

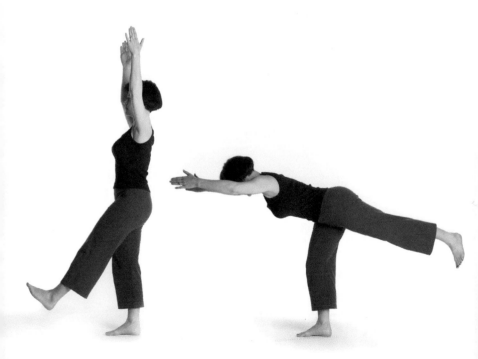

Half Moon Pose (Ardha Chandrasana) *Activating*

Half Moon is similar to Warrior III in that it is a fold from the hip, but in this pose you are challenging the core on the side of the body by opening up to the sky.

Begin this pose in Extended Side Angle Pose (Utthita Parsvakonasana). Start with the legs 3 to 4 feet apart. Turn the right foot out 90 degrees and the back foot in 45 degrees. Bend the right knee in line with the second toe, keeping the heel on the ground. Place the right forearm on the right knee and the back of the left hand on the low back.

To move into Half Moon, transfer your weight to the right foot so just the toe(s) of the back foot is on the ground. Place the right fingertips on the floor approximately 12 inches to the outside of the right foot. When you feel balanced, lift the left leg up off the floor and extend the right knee. Keep the body open and the head looking down toward the ground. To increase this challenge, extend the left arm to the sky and start to look forward or even up to the sky. Ensure the core is drawing up, there is energy flowing to the end of the left leg, and the chest is opening to the front. Allow the neck to rotate, but maintain its alignment with the thoracic spine. Hold this pose for 4 to 12 breaths, then repeat on the other side.

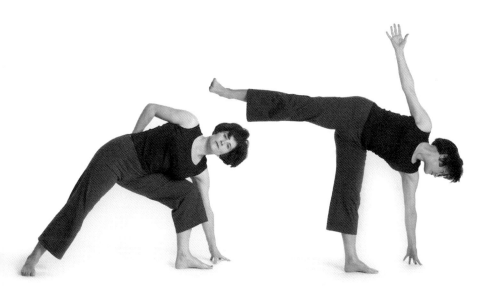

Plank Pose and Variations *Activating*

The Plank Pose increases the challenge to the inner core, specifically the transversus abdominis. To maintain the drawn-up position, the inner core must also draw up and hold in the abdominal contents. If the transversus abdominis (in combination with the internal and external obliques) does not have the strength to maintain alignment, the lower back arch will deepen and collapse, and you will feel the work transfer to the low back (specifically the erector spinae muscles). If this happens, discontinue the pose immediately because the likelihood of injury increases significantly if continued improperly. Adapt the exercise by lowering the intensity or decreasing the length of time in the pose until you are able to build up more strength with proper technique.

Start on your hands and knees, with your weight evenly spaced between your left and right sides and your hands under the shoulders (Table Pose). Draw up the inner core and then extend one leg behind you, keeping your toes on the floor. Without changing your body position (do not let either hip drop), extend the other leg to meet it. Hold this position for 4 to 12 breaths.

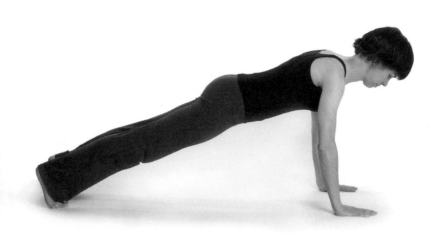

Please note, this is also a shoulder girdle stabilizer. Maintain the alignment of the shoulder blades against the spine as you do when you are standing in Mountain Pose. If the shoulder blades move to the side, you are overcontracting your chest muscles – try to open the collarbones on the inhale. Also make sure the shoulder blades do not collapse together or creep up into your ears. Any movement of the shoulder blades may indicate a weakness in your shoulder girdle muscles, which will be strengthened with good alignment in this pose. Lower the intensity of this pose until you can do it with stable shoulder blades.

For those with very strong upper abdominals, sometimes there is a tendency to overcontract the rectus abdominis (upper abdominals), creating a rounded upper spine. Increase the drawing in from the inner core and pelvis, and lengthen the upper spine on the inhale to balance this out.

Variations (increasing in intensity with each variation):
1. If your wrists are tight or injured, then this pose can be done from your elbows or forearms.

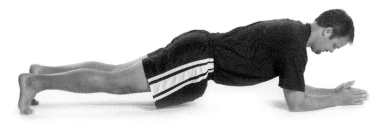

2. Extend the legs one at a time into full Plank, but then bring the knees to the floor, keeping your spinal alignment.

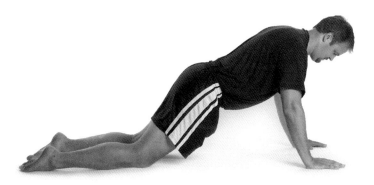

3. Lift one foot off the ground without allowing the hips to rock or drop.

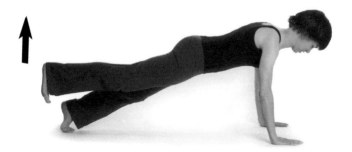

4. Lift the left foot off the ground and abduct it approximately 2 feet to the left, increasing the challenge for the obliques.

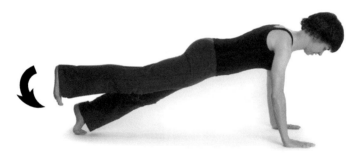

5. Lift one arm off the ground and extend it in front of you or out to the side. Start with the legs farther apart, and with time, move them closer together. Keep the pelvis still and the shoulder girdle neutral. Feel the increased activation in the internal and external obliques.

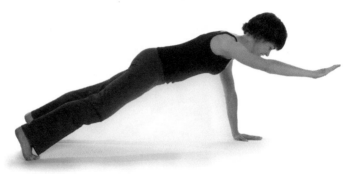

6. Rotate the body to the side so you are balancing on your right arm and right foot.

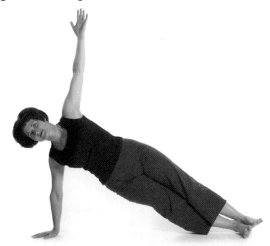

7. In the side plank position, lift the top leg and maintain the long line through the lower hip and waist. This position will increase the intensity and stability in the lower hip.

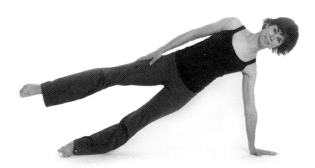

Nothing is so strong as gentleness, and nothing is so gentle as real strength.

– Ralph W. Sockman

The Stability Ball
and the Core

Relax your fingers.

Relax your hand.

Relax your heart.

Relax into a slower space, where

stakes are by definition lower.

– Maureen Killoran

The Stability Ball and the Core

A stability ball can be used as a prop to ease the depth of yoga poses or as a focal point to help you stay focused in the present. The instability aspect of the ball can also make the poses more challenging.

Stability ball key points:
- Stability ball training has been used by physical therapists for more than 50 years as a means of rehabilitating injuries. As a yoga prop, the ball adds balance challenges and helps your body learn to work as an integrated unit while performing movements.
- The correct ball height places the hips slightly above the knees when you sit on the ball.
- Always start with a wide base of support, then move to a narrow base of support once you feel confident in your position and to increase the challenge (e.g., start with arms out to the sides when feet are on the ball or legs wide when sitting on the ball).
- Work the poses slowly and gradually (incorporating more and more stability and balance work) to ensure you feel comfortable and safe.

Yoga key point:
- Connect with your breath, and increase your mind–body connection. This will help prevent injury and help you learn to honour your body and the place you are at right now. It will also help quiet the mind, relax the body, and empower the movement.

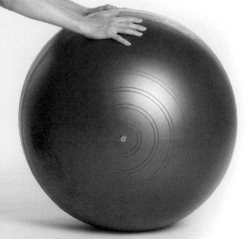

Lying Postures

Neck and Shoulder Release *Releasing*

a) Lie on your back, with your lower legs resting on the ball. Feel your breath.

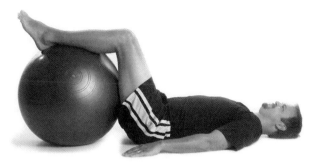

On an exhale, let your head drop to the side, releasing the ear to the floor. On an inhale, let the head float up, returning to neutral. Once the motion has been activated and the connection between the breath and the neck developed, activate the inner core to a level 3 out of 10, keeping the pelvis still.

Feel the release in the neck, the connection to the core, the breath, and the stable body. Explore the inner core/movement connection. Activate the core on the exhale and release on the inhale. Feel the change in your ability to stay stable as well as the depth of release in your neck.

b) Keeping the head and spine neutral, lift the right arm to the sky and over your head on the inhale, opening the ribs but keeping the pelvis and low ribs still. Exhale the arm back to your side. Repeat with the left arm. Feel the activation of the core stabilizing the spine, ribs, and pelvis while the arm and shoulder girdle move freely. Try to feel the opening of the ribs and the breath on the moving-arm side.

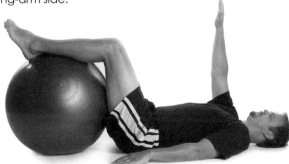

Little Bridge Pose (Setu Bandha Sarvangasana) *Activating*

Place your heels on top of the ball, knees and hips bent to 90 degrees. On your inhale, draw up from the base of your pelvis (inner core) as you peel your spine off the floor to the bottom of your shoulder blades. Release on your exhale.

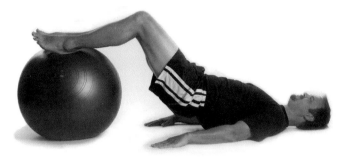

Note: It is harder to activate the inner core on the inhale, but it is important to develop this skill as well. The breath can be reversed, but the spine and rib opening will not be as deep.

Figure Four Hip Opener *Releasing*

Place your right heel on top of the ball and the ankle of the left leg just above the right knee. Keeping the spine neutral and stable, pull the right leg toward you (and thus the ball) until you feel a lengthening in the left hip.

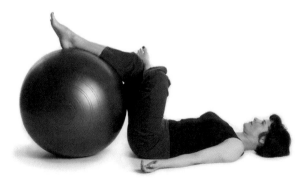

Feel your pelvis very stable and still (keep the tailbone on the floor – equal length through both sides of your waist). You are looking for a release in the hip, not a feeling of "stretch." Many times when we feel a stretch we are actually contracting or resisting the release. In this pose try to feel the release and allow the lengthening to happen. Be very aware of the alignment through the whole spine. *Does your head turn to the side when you open the hip?*

Kneeling Postures

Table Breathing *Breathing*
Kneel with your hands (or forearms if you have tight shoulders) on the ball.

Extend the ball away from you until you are creating a table with your body and arms. On your exhale, draw up from your inner core to the bottom of your ribs. Keep your spine neutral, and feel the stability around your spine.

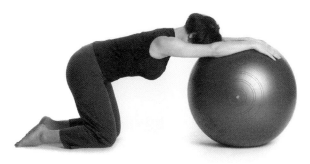

Cat Pose *Releasing*
In the same position as for Table breathing, add spinal movement to the breath and core activation, rolling up the spine from the pelvis to the shoulder blades. Inhale and lengthen the crown of the head from the tailbone.

Feel the articulation in each vertebra and the activation from the base of the pelvis up to the bottom of the ribs.

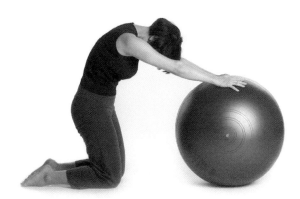

Kneeling Tadasana on the Ball *Activating*

Find a safe spot where you have space around you to roll off to the side or back and something in front of you to grab onto if you are about to roll forward. Holding onto something stable such as a countertop or wall to start, place your shins on the ball and come up to a tall kneeling position. Feel your inner core activate and the length through the spine all the way to the crown of the head. Feel the breath and the energy running up and down the spine.

When you feel comfortable, take your hands off your support (or maintain a very light grip). Eventually try bringing your arms over your head into a tall Mountain (Tadasana) position. Try to connect the inner core to the length in your spine, the relaxation in the shoulders, and the openness throughout the body. Feel which muscles need to activate (outer core) to stabilize you in this position.

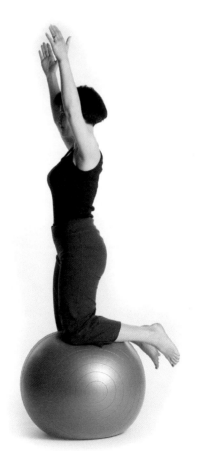

Shoulder Girdle Stabilization Postures/Ball to Belly Postures

Upward Facing Dog (Urdhva Mukha Svanasana) *Releasing*
Place the ball on your belly, still kneeling. Hands are just wider than shoulder width, on the side of the ball, down by your hips. Prepare by activating your core, then pull your shoulder blades slightly down your spine and rib cage, reaching your breastbone and heart forward and open. You can extend this pose by tucking the toes under and lengthening the legs behind you.

You are looking for a smooth, continuous curve throughout the whole spine, so if you feel this in one place in your back, you may be hyperextending this area in relation to the rest of the back. To prevent this, increase the activation in your lower core, trying to focus the extension through the thoracic spine. You may also have taken the pose too deep and need to back off.

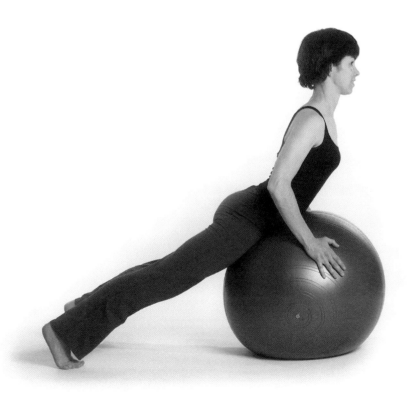

Plank Pose *Activating*

Place your belly on the ball, hands on the floor. Keeping your core activated, walk your hands out forward until you feel your shoulder girdle and outer core activated. (See Plank Pose in chapter 3 for key points to watch for.) Hold this position, increasing the activation of the inner core with each exhale.

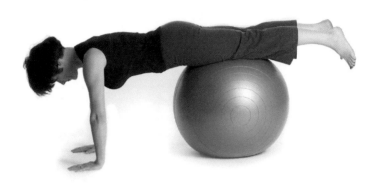

Downward Facing Dog (Adho Mukha Svanasana) into Handstand (Adho Mukha Vrksasana) *Activating*

In the previous Plank position, bend from the top of the thighs (not the spine) and reach your sit bones to the sky, coming into a pike position with the ball rolling along your shins.

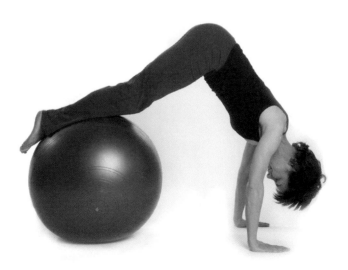

If you are far enough out, you may need to tuck your toes under and roll the ball onto your toes or the balls of your feet. As you increase your strength and roll up farther, you will eventually come to a vertical upper body position (handstand). Be sure to maintain a neutral low back alignment; do not allow the low back to round.

Neutral Alignment   **Rounded Back**

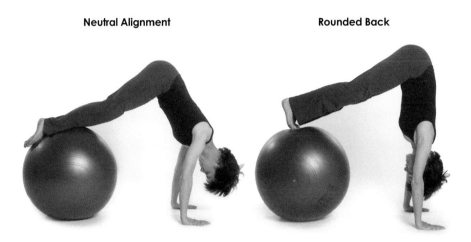

Experiment with your cervical alignment, and see if keeping your eyes on the ground vs. looking at the ball helps you maintain your neutral low back curve. Focus on bringing the diaphragm over the shoulder blades and feeling the connection between the shoulder blades, diaphragm, and pelvic floor/transverse abdominal muscles. Experiment with this interesting connection in your handstand without the ball.

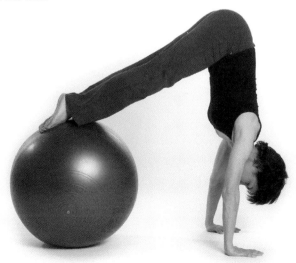

Seated Postures

Sitting on the Ball *Activating*

Sitting on the ball is similar in theory to standing on one leg. When you stand, you can feel your ankle and foot stabilizing you. When you sit on the ball, the outer and inner core stabilize you from moving. Start in a stable position (legs wide) and move to a smaller base of support (legs together or one leg on the ground, the other lifted up). Try various arm positions, or rotate the spine into a seated twist to feel the core activate to balance you.

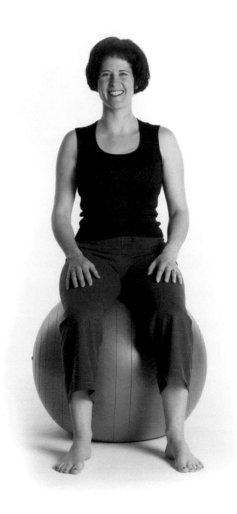

Eagle Pose (Garudasana) *Releasing*

Sitting on the ball, cross your right elbow over your left. Bend your elbows, and either bring your hands to your shoulders or wrap your wrists around each other. Bring your shoulder blades down your spine, elbows forward and up, and feel the opening between your shoulder blades. Let your head go to the place it needs to be (try turning the head, dropping the chin, and so on). You will feel the right place when you get there.

Try to relax and release the neck and shoulder girdle while the core stabilizes you from the ball up. You can add the leg lifted or crossed when you feel stable on the ball and are able to increase the activation in the core while still being able to release the neck, upper back, and shoulders.

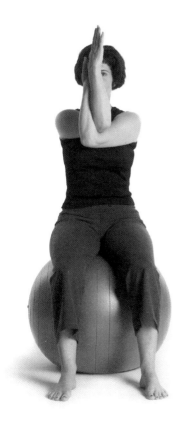
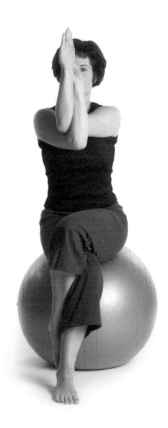

Bridge to Modified Bow *Activating*

Sit on the ball and roll down until the ball supports your head and shoulders, the knees are bent to 90 degrees, and the body forms an upward facing table. (Because you can't see the ball in this position, it involves trust in your ball and your abilities. You can place your fingertips on the floor beside you for reassurance, or you can always lower your buttocks to the floor if you want to come out of the pose.) Activate your core and feel the stability of your bridge/table. From here, bring your arms to the sky and then over your head. Extend your legs and let your heart open to the sky as you bend back over the ball. Feel the stability of the core, the openness of the chest, and the energy up your body.

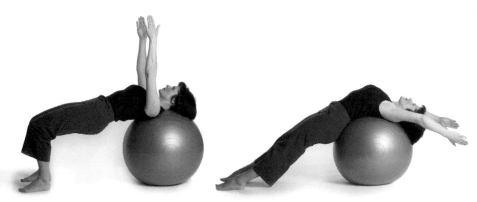

If you feel this pose in your low back or your neck is no longer supported, you are too high on the ball; come out and adjust your position so that your chest opens and your low back stays stable. Finish this pose by bending the spine forward and releasing the spine in the other direction.

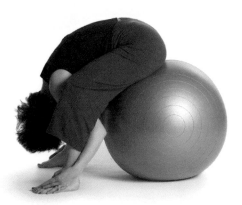

Warrior II Pose (Virabhadrasana II) *Releasing*

Sit on the ball with legs wide. Rotate your right knee and foot 90 degrees from your hip. Your right knee can bend up to 90 degrees, as long as it is both pain-free and aligned with hip and middle toes. Extend your left leg back straight, and rotate your heel out 30 to 45 degrees.

Activate your inner core and left buttock, ensuring the alignment of the right knee over the toe. Work to outwardly rotate both thighs, and feel the extension down into the ground with the outer arch of the left foot.

Feel the openness in the inner thigh and pelvis and the length through the crown of the head toward the sky. You can extend the arms over the legs, but keep the shoulders relaxed and the collarbones open. This is a strength pose – feel the energy flow through the body, through the lines down the legs, out the arms, and through the crown of the head. Feel the belief in yourself that you can defeat anything. You are the warrior!

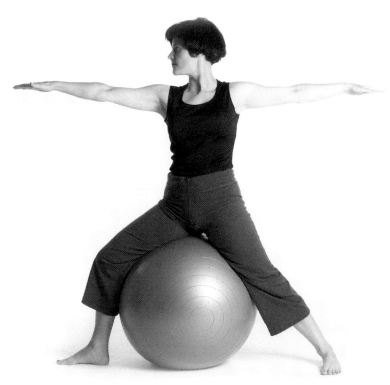

Warrior I Pose (Virabhadrasana I) *Releasing*

Warrior I is similar to Warrior II except you are now facing your front leg. Let the back heel rise up, and rotate the pelvis around to face the front and to be level and squared. Move the ball between the legs a little more than in Warrior II so that you can press your back thigh into the ball and feel the front of the hip open. Extend the back foot toward the ground, but keep the heel lifted and focus on the thigh instead of the calf. Activate the inner core, and feel the stability in the pelvis and the bottom ribs drawn down to the front hips. Your pelvis may tilt anteriorly, but try to minimize this by stabilizing with your inner core, thereby keeping the opening in the hip instead of the low back.

Raise your arms over your head, and allow your chest to open as if you are running across the finish line. Feel both the opening through the front of your body and the length in the back of your body. You are now not only the warrior but also able to receive what is being delivered to you.

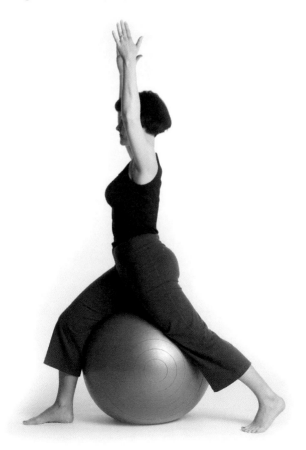

The BOSU Balance Trainer, Foam Roller, or Body Weight

Tension is who you think you should be. Relaxation is who you are.

– Chinese Proverb

The BOSU Balance Trainer, Foam Roller, or Body Weight

The BOSU (BOth Sides Up) Balance Trainer and the foam roller give proprioceptive (sense of the body's positioning) feedback to help you feel if you are losing your stability and core activation. These props also increase the challenge and help you identify if other muscles are taking over.

Keep the mind in the body, and watch how the whole body reacts to each position you take it through. *Are there some positions in which it is harder to activate your core? Do you find yourself holding your breath in some positions in order to hold your core in? Can you find the softness and the stability in each pose?* It is this awareness that is yoga.

You can try all the following exercises without a BOSU Balance Trainer or foam roller and still benefit and feel challenged.

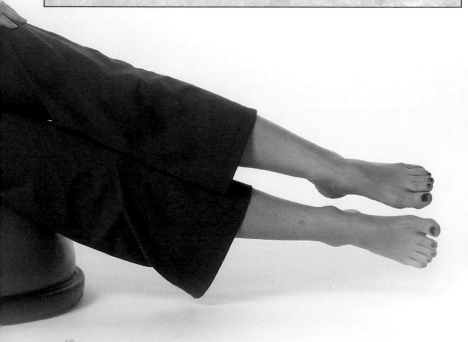

Swimming Locust (Salabhasana) on the BOSU Balance Trainer

Activating

Lying on your tummy on the BOSU Balance Trainer, extend your arms and legs out. Activate your core and draw the belly up and away from the "bubble," as if you are trying to lie very lightly on it. Lift one leg off the ground without moving the low back or rocking on the bubble. Release and repeat with the other leg. Make sure you are not holding your breath; breathe into the side back ribs while the core is being activated.

Increase the challenge in the following ways:
  • Lift one arm with the opposite leg.

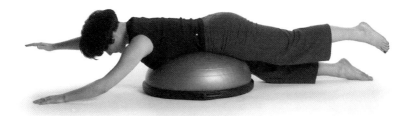

  • Hover all limbs off the ground as a starting position, then alternate lifting one leg and one arm.

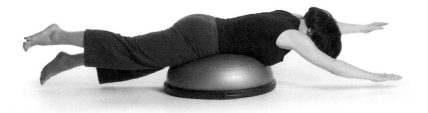

  • Increase the speed of the movements without the torso moving on the bubble.
  • Turn your thumbs up to increase activation of the lower and middle trapezius.

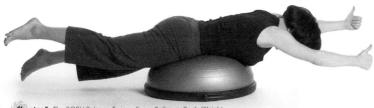

Side Plank on the BOSU Balance Trainer *Activating*

Lying sideways on the BOSU Balance Trainer, place your hip on top of the bubble and your lower arm on the floor, bent 90 degrees at the elbow. Ensure that the elbow is directly below the shoulder. Lengthen the neck and release any tension in the shoulder and neck area. Lift your legs off the floor to create one long line from your crown to your toes. If you cannot lift your legs off the ground, move higher up on the bubble; if it is too easy or you feel tension in the neck and shoulders, move lower (it may be the difference of an inch or even less). Pull your inner core up, and feel the activation of the lower waist (internal and external obliques). Try to keep the hips and shoulders stacked.

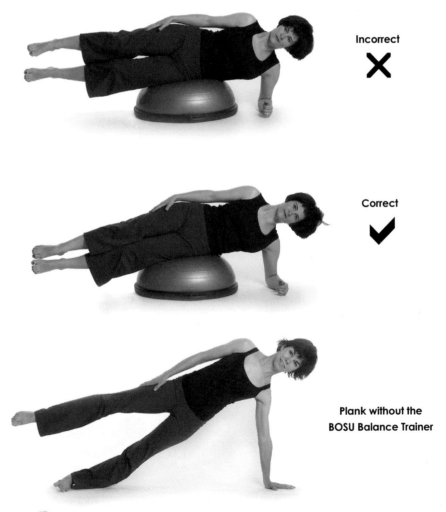

Incorrect
✘

Correct
✔

Plank without the
BOSU Balance Trainer

Variations (increasing in intensity with each variation):

1. Lift the top leg up as high as you can go without moving the pelvis or rotating the front of the leg upward (about 30 degrees), then lower to the opposite leg (or neutral alignment).

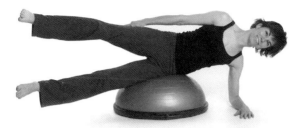

2. Move the top leg back into hip extension, then stay in this position without losing your stability on the BOSU Balance Trainer, without losing pelvic stability, and without increasing shoulder girdle and neck tension.

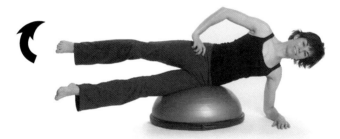

3. Keeping the torso still, bring the top leg forward on the inhale and behind you on the exhale. Be sure to move only through your hip's active range of motion rather than rounding your back when you come forward and hyperextending the back as you reach behind you. Feel the leg reaching away from you. The stabilization of the spine will increase the activation of the multifidi in your back.

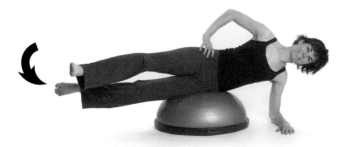

Kneeling Tadasana on the BOSU Balance Trainer *Activating*

Place your shins on the BOSU Balance Trainer and come up to a tall position. Feel your inner core activate. Feel the length through the spine all the way to the crown of the head. Feel the breath and the energy running up and down the spine.

Bring your arms over your head into a tall Mountain (Tadasana) position. Try to connect the inner core to the length in your spine, the relaxation in the shoulders, and the openness throughout the body. Feel which muscles need to activate (outer core) to stabilize you in this position.

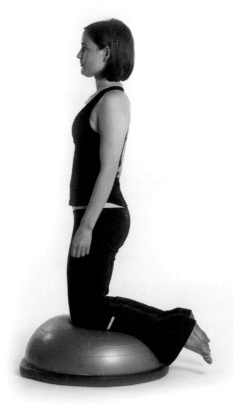

This is also a great exercise on the stability ball or on the roller – just make sure that when you do it on the ball, you have space around you to roll off to the side or back and something in front of you to grab onto if you are about to roll forward (see chapter 4).

Marching Abdominals on the Roller *Activating*

As described in chapter 1.

Start by lying on your back lengthwise on the roller, with your knees bent and feet flat on the floor. Keep your arms on the floor for support, but release your shoulders (do not press into the ground with your hands). Lift one foot off the ground approximately 1 to 4 inches (just take its weight off the floor), and see if you can maintain a stable, nonrocking pelvis (and roller). Lower the leg to the ground and repeat on the other side. Keep changing legs, ensuring there is no rocking or dropping of the pelvis when you lift or lower the foot. The roller will give you increased feedback – try to keep the roller still.

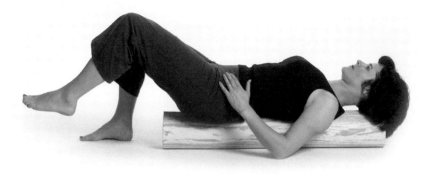

Eventually progress to only your fingertips on the ground, to hands across your belly (elbows out so you can stop yourself from moving far if you do start to roll), to hands across your chest, to hands above your head (lower ribs connected to your pelvis through your inner core).

Leg Circles on the Roller *Activating*

Start by lying on your back lengthwise on the roller, with your knees bent and feet flat on the floor. Hands can start on the floor, but try not to press into the hands (place only your fingertips on the floor or turn the palms toward you, allowing only the outer side of the hand to be in contact with the floor).

Activate your inner core and lengthen one leg toward the ceiling (i.e., to where the knee can go straight – if this causes your hip flexors to grab, your leg to shake, or an uncomfortable feeling in your hamstrings, then gently bend the knee). Slide the other leg out along the ground as far as you can without the pelvis changing. Draw small circles on the ceiling, keeping the pelvis still and stable (remember that glass of red wine?). Keep the knee, ankle, and toes still so you are moving from your hip.

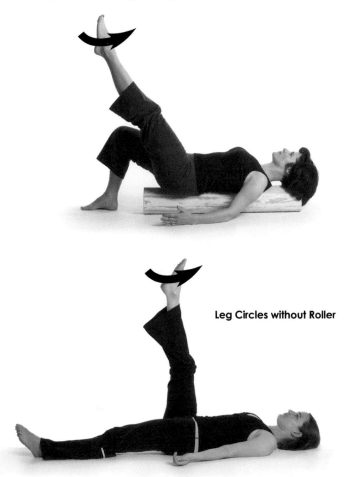

Leg Circles without Roller

Cobra Pose (Bhujangasana) with the Roller *Activating*

Lying on your tummy, place your hands on the roller, with your arms extended over your head. Feel the legs lengthened toward the back wall, while keeping the toes on the floor. Initiate the movement by drawing up your inner core and moving your shoulder blades down the spine.

Peel your chest off the floor as if you are pressing away a marble with your chest. Keep the back of the neck long, without any creases (look just slightly in front of you). Come up only as high as you can with the mobility of the back (don't press into the hands on the roller). This position can produce increased mobility and activation in the upper back muscles and a feeling of openness in the chest, with a stable and connected inner core.

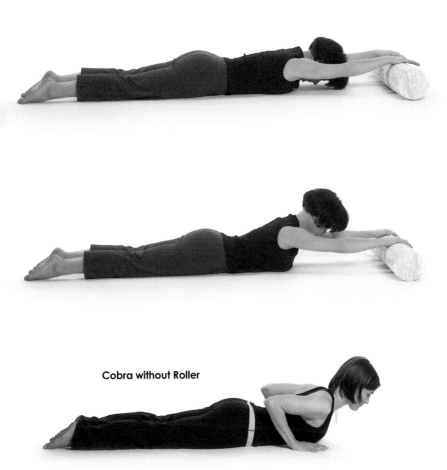

Cobra without Roller

The body is your temple. Keep it pure and clean for the soul to reside in.

– B.K.S. Iyengar

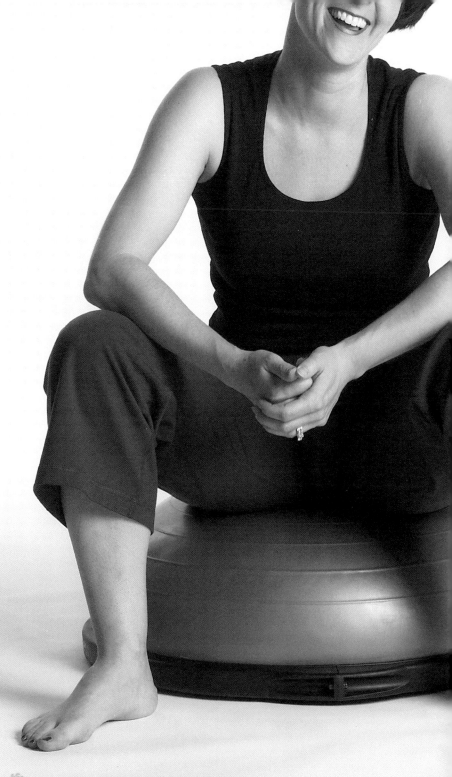

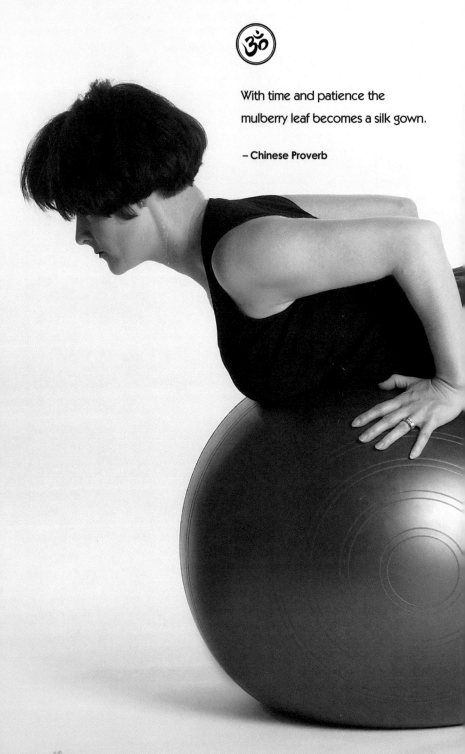

ॐ

With time and patience the
mulberry leaf becomes a silk gown.

– Chinese Proverb

Putting Stability into Practice

The universe is full of magical
things patiently waiting for
our wits to grow sharper.

– Eden Phillpotts

Putting Stability into Practice

This book is designed to teach you about the inner core – how to find it, how to activate it, and how to strengthen and challenge it. It is, however, only the beginning. Once you have connected with your inner core, you need to apply what you have learned to every pose you practice in yoga as well as everyday activities and movements. Find out for yourself how the inner core is related to a pose and what influence it has. Think of it as on a dial from 0 to 10. At what level does it need to be involved? Sometimes it needs to stand back and be the stagehand, sometimes the director, sometimes the supporting actor, sometimes the leading role. Learn how to make your inner core functional, then watch the strength and release that happens throughout the rest of your body. To make things happen, you need to develop a plan and know when to move to the next level so you can progress effectively, positively, and safely.

Start with level 1, and when you have achieved the key points, move to level 2. You can try level 2 before all the points are achieved, but make sure your technique in level 2 poses incorporates what you have learned from level 1 (most important: core activation; pelvic and shoulder girdle stability). Do the same when you would like to try level 3.

You may also find that some poses in level 2 are easier for you than some of the level 1 poses; this occurs because of your strengths and weaknesses, so please use this level system as a guide only. Always listen to your body first.

Keep in mind the progression notes on stability, and try incorporating little changes to the poses you are becoming comfortable with to slowly increase the challenge (see chapter 3).

Consult a physiotherapist or a certified yoga or Pilates instructor if you are having difficulty ensuring your technique is correct.

Level 1 – Increasing Awareness and Activation
Key points: increased awareness of the inner core and how to activate it; level and non-rocking pelvis with hip and knee release and marching abdominals

Breathing poses:
- Belly breathing – chapter 1, page 26
- Crocodile breathing – chapter 1, page 27
- Table breathing on ball – chapter 4, page 63

Release poses:
- Neck and shoulder release – chapter 4, page 61
- Figure four hip opener on ball – chapter 4, page 62
- Cat with ball – chapter 4, page 63

Activation poses:
- Drawing up – chapter 1, page 29 and 30
- Standing leg circles – chapter 1, page 33
- Marching abdominals – chapter 1, page 34
- Hip and knee release – chapter 1, page 35
- Table – chapter 1, page 36
- Mountain – chapter 3, page 49
- Sitting on the ball – chapter 4, page 68

The more you focus on breath and awareness, the faster you will improve.

Level 2 – Increasing Strength

Key points: inner core maintains connection and activation in each pose; pelvis is able to maintain neutral alignment; shoulders and neck area are able to stay relaxed; increased strength in waist (obliques) vs. belly popping out (rectus abdominis or loss of activation of transversus); Plank on elbows and toes feels stable for at least six breaths (approximately 30 seconds)

Release poses (including some activation):
- Eagle on ball – chapter 4, page 69

Activation poses:
- Half Moon – chapter 3, page 53
- Warrior III – chapter 3, page 52
- Tree – chapter 3, page 50
- Plank from knees – chapter 3, page 54
- Plank using elbows – chapter 3, page 55
- Side Plank – chapter 3, page 57
- Little Bridge on ball – chapter 4, page 62
- Plank on ball – chapter 4, page 66
- Bridge to modified Bow – chapter 4, page 70
- Butterfly – chapter 5, Bookmark
- Marching abdominals on roller with hands on the ground – chapter 5, page 79
- Marching abdominals on roller with fingertips on the ground – chapter 5, page 79
- Cobra with roller – chapter 5, page 81
- Kneeling Tadasana on BOSU Balance Trainer – chapter 5, page 78
- Side Plank on BOSU® Balance Trainer variation 1 – chapter 5, page 77
- Side Plank on BOSU® Balance Trainer, variation 2 – chapter 5, page 77
- Side Plank on BOSU® Balance Trainer, variation 3 – chapter 5, page 77
- Swimming Locust on BOSU® Balance Trainer, lifting one leg – chapter 5, page 75
- Swimming Locust on BOSU® Balance Trainer, lifting one arm – chapter 5, page 75
- Swimming Locust on BOSU® Balance Trainer, lifting one arm and opposite leg – chapter 5, page 75
- Swimming Locust on BOSU® Balance Trainer, hovering with alternating arm and leg – chapter 5, page 75
- Swimming Locust on BOSU® Balance Trainer, increasing the fluttering of arms and legs – chapter 5, page 75
- Swimming Locust on BOSU® Balance Trainer, turning thumbs up – chapter 5, page 75

Level 3 – Challenging Your Strength and Stability
Key points: stability against increased speed of movement; increased strength with longer levers; able to maintain activation of inner core with increased activation of outer core; shoulder girdle relaxed.

Release poses (including activation):
- Warrior I on ball – chapter 4, page 72
- Warrior II on ball – chapter 4, page 71
- Upward Facing Dog on ball – chapter 4, page 65

Activation poses:
- Plank, lifting one foot – chapter 3, page 56
- Plank, lifting one foot and abducting – chapter 3, page 56
- Plank, lifting one arm – chapter 3, page 56
- Downward Facing Dog on ball – chapter 4, page 66
- Handstand on the ball – chapter 4, page 67
- Kneeling Tadasana on ball – chapter 4, page 64
- Marching abdominals on roller with hands across belly – chapter 5, page 79
- Marching abdominals on roller with hands across chest – chapter 5, page 79
- Marching abdominals on roller with hands above head – chapter 5, page 79
- Leg circles on roller – chapter 5, page 80
- Side Plank on on BOSU® Balance Trainer, variation 1, increasing the speed to a flutter – chapter 5, page 77
- Swimming Locust on on BOSU® Balance Trainer, hovering with alternating arm and leg – chapter 5, page 75
- Swimming Locust on on BOSU® Balance Trainer, increasing the fluttering of arms and legs – chapter 5, page 75
- Swimming Locust on on BOSU® Balance Trainer, turning thumbs up – chapter 5, page 75

Creating Your Plan:

- Start with at least one breathing pose and one activation pose.
- Include releasing poses for postural muscles that need to be released or lengthened at the beginning and interspersed within your program (see a yoga therapist or physiotherapist for a personalized program that assesses and meets your needs).
- Add as many stability-creating poses as you have time for.
- Come out of a pose or move onto the next pose if any of the following occur:
  - a. Your body tension increases and you start to lose your inner core activation.
  - b. Your breath starts to increase in speed, or you hold your breath.
  - c. Your mind wanders off into the past or the future.
- Finish with one or more of the following relaxation techniques:
  - a. Lie flat and bring your mind into your body. Notice any changes (release any judgment as to what you should feel – just watch for any differences).
  - b. Count your breath backward from 20.
  - c. Listen to Suzette's *Savasana: A Guided Relaxation* CD.

See the sample plan on the following page for an example of how your plan may develop.

Approximate Time Chart and Sample Plan

Level 1 – increasing awareness and activation
Total time: approximately 25 min

STEP 1	STEP 2	STEP 3	STEP 4
Warm-Up	**Releasing Poses**	**Stability Poses**	**Relaxation**
Diaphragm breathing: 3 min	Neck and shoulder release with ball: 2 min	Standing leg circles: 2 min	Listen to track one of *Savasana*: 9 min
Hip release: 2 min	Figure four hip opener on ball: 4 min	Marching abdominals: 2 min	

Level 2 – increasing strength
Total time: approximately 30 min

STEP 1	STEP 2	STEP 3	STEP 4
Warm-Up	**Releasing Poses**	**Stability Poses**	**Relaxation**
Crocodile breathing: 3 min	Neck and shoulder release with ball: 2 min	Tree: 4 min	Listen to track two of *Savasana*: 16 min
Marching abdominals: 2 min	Cat with ball: 1 min	Plank from knees: 2 min	
		Side Plank: 2 min	

Level 3 – challenging your strength and stability
Total time: approximately 30 min

STEP 1	STEP 2	STEP 3	STEP 4
Warm-Up	**Releasing Poses**	**Stability Poses**	**Relaxation**
Table breathing: 2 min	Warrior I & II on ball: 5 min	Downward Facing Dog on ball: 3 min	Listen to track three of *Savasana*: 16 min
Cat with ball: 1 min		Swimming Locust on BOSU Balance Trainer: 2 min	

Yoga for the Core: Finding Stability in an Unstable Environment

Name _____

Date at start of program _____

Rate your awareness of the core:
None 1 2 3 4 5 High
Rate your ability to keep the spine and pelvis level during
the hip and knee release pose:
Not Able 1 2 3 4 5 Very Able
Rate your pain or discomfort level (average over the past week):
None 1 2 3 4 5 6 7 8 9 10 Unbearable

In the chart below, please check a box for each day you do your
Yoga for the Core plan.

	SUN	MON	TUES	WED	THURS	FRI	SAT	Comments
Week 1								
Week 2								
Week 3								
Week 4								

Date at end of program _____

Rate your awareness of the core:
None 1 2 3 4 5 High
Rate your ability to keep the spine and pelvis level during
the hip and knee release pose:
Not Able 1 2 3 4 5 Very Able
Rate your pain or discomfort level (average over the past week):
None 1 2 3 4 5 6 7 8 9 10 Unbearable

Comment on how you feel the Yoga for the Core stability program
has affected your pain or your ability to perform daily activities:

_____

_____

_____

_____

_____

_____

_____

_____

"I honour the place
within you where the entire
Universe resides.

I honour the place within you
of love, light, truth, and peace.
I honour the place within you
where, when you are in that place
in you and I am in that place in
me, there is only One of us."

Namaste

References

Bogduk, Nikolai. 1997. *Clinical Anatomy of the Lumbar Spine and Sacrum.* 3rd edition. New York: Churchill Livingstone.

Dürckheim, Karlfried Graf. 2004. *Hara: The Vital Center of Man.* UK: George Allen and Unwin.

Evans, Meaghan. 2006. *Exercising Your Pelvic Floor: Part 1 & 2.* Calgary Health Region Pelvic Floor Clinic. Women's Health Resources.

Farhi, Donna. 1996. *The Breathing Book.* New York: Holt.

Gray, Henry. 1985. *Anatomy: Descriptive and Surgical.* 15th edition. London: Chancellor Press.

Hately Aldous, Susi. 2004. *Anatomy and Asana: Preventing Yoga Injuries.* Calgary: Functional Synergy Press.

Iyengar, BKS. 2005. Light on Life: *The Yoga Journey to Wholeness, Inner Peace and Ultimate Freedom.* USA Rodale Inc.

Janda, V. 1983. *Muscle Function Testing.* London: Butterworths.

Kapit, Wynn, and Lawrence M. Elson. 1993. *The Anatomy Coloring Book.* 2nd edition. New York: Harper Collins.

Richardson, Carolyn, Paul W. Hodges, and Julie Hides. 2004. *Therapeutic Exercise for Lumbopelvic Stabilization: A Motor Control Approach for the Treatment and Prevention of Low Back Pain.* London: Churchill Livingstone.

STOTT PILATES. 2001. Comprehensive Matwork. Merrithew Corporation. Wallden, Matthew James. July 2004. *The Core: Part 2.* Available: www.ptonthenet.com.

Woodruff, Dianne. Dec. 3, 2002. *Postural and Phasic Muscles.* Available: www.ptonthenet.com.

Index

Index

Breath
    yoga vs. pilates, 28
Breath awareness, 10
    connecting with movement, 10
    connecting with neck, 61
    with improvement of core stability,
    12
Breath counting, backwards from 20,
    90
Breath focus, as key to improvement,
    87
Breathing poses, 8
    for awareness enhancement, 87
    belly breathing, 26
    crocodile breathing, 27
    importance in yoga plan, 90
    Table breathing on ball, 63
Breathing rate, increases in, 90
Bridge pose, to modified Bow, 70
    as strength-enhancing activation
    pose, 88
Bulbospongiosus, 29
Butterfly pose, 88

C

Cat pose with ball, 43, 63, 91
    as release pose, 87
Cervical spine
    maintaining neutral alignment in, 42
    proper alignment in Handstand, 67
Change, ability to withstand
    (dvandvanabhighatah), 38
Chest press, and inner core
    dysfunction, 25
Childbirth, and inner core dysfunction,
    25
Clam pose, 41
Cobra pose (Bhujangasana),
    with roller, 81
    as strength-enhancing activation
    pose, 88
Cohen, Bonnie Bainbridge, 105
Compensating movements
    dangers of destabilization, 39
    identifying and releasing, 7
    minimizing in smaller joints, 11
Core
    benefits of promoting health in, 7
    as center of balance and root of
    movements, 7
    as hara, 7
    Hawaiian interpretation of, 7
    spine as, 11
Core muscles
    postural muscles as, 19
    strengthening and lengthening, 19
Correct technique, 86
Crocodile breathing, 27, 91
    for awareness enhancement, 87

D

Deconditioning, and inner core

dysfunction, 25
Deltoid, posterior, 23, 24
Diaphragm
    attachment to low back, 26, 27
    connection to pelvic floor, 30
    crocodile breathing exercise, 27
    in inner core, 25
    physiology, 26
Diaphragm breathing, 19, 91
    emotional response from, 27
Downward Facing Dog pose (Adha
    Mukha Svanasana), on ball, 66, 91
    as strength- and stability-
    challenging pose, 89
Drawing up pose, 31
    as activation pose, 87
Durckheim, Karlfried Graf, 17

E

Eagle pose on ball, 43, 69
    as strength-enhancing release
    pose, 88
Eight principles of movement, 9. See
    also Movement
    adopt relaxed resilience, 13
    breathing while boosting core
    stability, 12
    connect spinal movement with
    large joints, 11
    initiate movement, 11
    less is more, 15
    move in pain-free range of motion,
    14
    move joints in optimum range of
    motion, 12
    nourish relaxation, 10
Energy transformation, breathing for,
    28
Erector spinae, 22
Exercise ball, 8
Exercise equipment, improper use and
    inner core dysfunction, 25
Exhalation, on spinal flexion, 28
External anal sphincter, 29
External oblique, 21, 23, 24
External stimuli, reacting to, for stability
    challenge, 47
External urethral orifice, 29

F

Fast-twitch fibers, in phasic muscles, 18
Figure four hip opener on ball, 62, 91
    as release pose, 87
Fitness ball, pelvic floor exercises with,
    30
Foam roller, 63–74
    Cobra pose on, 81
    leg circles on, 80
    Marching Abdominals on, 79
Forcing, vs. relaxed resilience, 13
Functional Synergy
    contact information, 103

Index

eight principles of movement, 8, 10
history and purpose, 103
less is more principle at, 15

G

Gastrocnemius, 22
Gastrointestinal tract infection, and
inner core dysfunction, 25
Gentleness, 58
Gluten intolerance, and inner core
dysfunction, 25
Gluteus maximus, 23, 24, 29, 41
Gluteus medius, 21, 23, 24
Gluteus minimus, 21, 24
Gracilis, 20, 22

H

Half Moon pose (Ardha
Chandrasana), 53
as strength-enhancing activation
pose, 88
Handstand pose (Adho Mukha
Vrksasana), on ball, 67
as strength- and stability-
challenging pose, 89
Hara, as core, 7
Hatha yoga, 28
Head support exercise, 42
Hip abduction, 39
pressing into strap exercise, 40
Hip adduction, 39
Hip and knee injury, due to weak inner
core, 25
Hip and knee release, 35
as activation pose, 87
Hip flexors, 40
in Clam pose, 41
releasing during outer core
exercises, 39–41
Hip joint, avoiding compensating
movements with tight, 12
Hip release, 91
Hips
bending from, 29
cultivating pure movement at, 11
external rotators, 41
Holding breath, 90
Hyperextension, avoiding in Upward
Facing Dog pose, 65

I

Iliopsoas, 20, 39
Inhalation, initiating pelvic floor
muscles on, 28
Initiate movement principle, 11
Injury
avoiding by increasing stability, 46
customized yoga programs for, 103
due to weak inner core, 25
inner and outer core use to
prevent, 36

phasic muscles' susceptibility to, 19
preventing during yoga, 15
preventing with proper breathing,
12
reactiveness of phasic muscles to,
18
Inner core, 17, 86
activating through abdominal
bracing vs. hollowing, 36
activating using different postures,
33
anterior pelvic floor in, 25
diaphragm in, 25
increased awareness of, 87
maintaining connection and
activation while increasing
strength, 88
multifidi in, 25
muscles involved in, 25
pelvic and spinal stability with, 25
postural muscles as, 19
relation to specific poses, 86
stabilizing through, 33
transversus abdominis in, 25
Inner core dysfunction, reasons for, 25
Inner thigh, opening in Warrior II pose,
71
Intent, aligning with movement, 105
Intercostal muscles, 26
Internal obliques, 21, 24
Ischiocavernosus, 29
Isometric exercises, 19
Isotonic exercises, 19
Iyengar, BKS, 16, 82

J

Jaw tightening, 14

K

Kneeling Tadasana, with BOSU
Balance Trainer, 78
as strength-enhancing activation
pose, 88
Kraftsow, Gary, 38

L

Large joints
connecting spinal movement with,
11
role in relaxed resilience, 13
Latissimus dorsi, 23, 24
Leg circles, on roller, 80
as strength- and stability-
challenging pose, 89
Leg press, and inner core dysfunction,
25
Levator ani, 29
Levator scapulae, 22
Lever lengths, increasing for stability
challenge, 47
Lightness (angalaghavam), 38

Index

Little Bridge pose (Setu Bandha
  Sarvangasana), 34
  on ball, 62
    as strength-enhancing
      activation pose, 88
Longus capitis, 21, 24
Longus colli, 21, 24
Low back, improperly stabilizing
  with hip muscles, 39
Low back pain
  due to weak inner core, 25
  and inner core dysfunction, 25
  preventing with Table pose during
    pregnancy, 36
Lower belly, as source of strength, 44
Lower rib cage, Pilates breathing
  into, 28
Lower vertebrae, hypermobility as
  compensation, 12

M

Marching abdominals, 34, 91
  as activation pose, 87
  on roller with fingertips on
    ground, 79
    as strength-enhancing
      activation pose, 88
  on roller with hands above
    head, 79
    as strength- and stability-
      challenging pose, 89
  on roller with hands across
    belly, 79
    as strength- and stability-
      challenging pose, 89
  on roller with hands across
    chest, 79, 89
  on roller with hands on
    ground, 79, 88
    as strength-enhancing
      activation pose, 88
Mind wandering, 90
Mountain pose (Tadasana), 49
  as activation pose, 87
Movement
  aligning attention and intent
    with, 105
  avoiding and releasing
    compensating, 7
  connecting breath awareness
    with, 10
  coordinating spinal and large-
    joint, 11
  core as root of, 7
  eight principles of, 9–15
  fluidity within, 4
  increasing complexity for
    stability challenge, 47
  outer core muscles and, 19
  in pain-free range of motion, 14
Mula bandha, 7. See also Pelvic floor
  lock (mula bandha)

Multifidi, 22
  contraction exercise, 32
  in inner core, 25
  physiology of, 32
  stabilizing in Marching Abdominals
    pose, 34
  Standing leg circles exercise for, 33
Muscle fatigue, 14
Muscle shortening, by postural
  muscles under stress, 19
Muscle tension. See also Body tension
  decreasing by strengthening core,
    7
Muscles. See Phasic muscles;
  Postural muscles

N

Na'au (gut), 7
Neck and shoulder release, 61, 87
  with ball, 91
  Cat pose with ball for, 43, 63
  diaphragmatic breathing for, 43
  in Eagle pose, 69
  Eagle pose on ball for, 43, 69
  exercises for, 43
  head support exercise, 42
Neck and shoulder tension
  avoiding during inner core
    exercises, 33
  due to weak inner core, 25
Neck and shoulders, keeping relaxed
  during strength-enhancing poses, 88
Neck tightening, 14
  reducing during hip and knee
    release, 35
Neutral alignment, with strength-
  enhancing poses, 88
Nourish relaxation principle, 10

O

Obliques, increasing strength in, 88
Okada, Master, 44
Optimum range of motion, moving
  joints in, 12
Outer core, 17
  phasic muscles and, 19
  releasing helper muscles in, 37–39

P

Pain, distinguishing between types
  of, 14
Pain-free range of motion principle, 14
Pectoralis major, 20, 21, 24
  as secondary respiratory muscle, 26
Pelvic diaphragm, 29–31
Pelvic floor lock (mula bandha), 28.
  See also Mula bandha
Pelvic floor muscles, 29–31
  connection to diaphragm, 30
  initiating on inhalation, 28
  in inner core, 25

Index

Index

Proprioceptive feedback, with BOSU Balance Trainer, 74

Q

Quadratus lumborum, 20, 22

R

Range of motion (ROM), moving joints in optimum, 12
Rectum control, improving through pelvic floor muscles, 29
Rectus abdominis, 21, 24
  controlling in strength-enhancing poses, 88
Rectus femoris, 20, 22, 39
Relaxation
  within action, 4
  nourishing, 10
Relaxation poses
  including in yoga plan, 90
  time charts and sample plans, 91
Relaxed resilience principle, 13
Release poses, 8
  for awareness enhancement and activation, 87
  Cat with ball, 63, 87
  for challenging strength and stability, 89
  Eagle on ball, 69, 88
  Figure four hip opener on ball, 62, 87
  Neck and shoulder release, 61, 87
  for strength enhancement, 88
  time chart and sample plans, 91
  Upward Facing Dog on ball, 65, 89
  Warrior I on ball, 72, 89
  Warrior II on ball, 71, 89
Repetitive strain injuries (RSI), due to weak inner core, 25
Resistance, increasing for stability challenge, 47
Rhomboids, 23, 24
Root chakra, 7
Rotators, 22

S

Sacroiliac joint
  avoiding bending from, 29
  hypermobility as compensation, 12
SAID training principle, 46
Sample plan, 90-92
Savasana: A Guided Relaxation, 90, 91
Scalenus, 21, 24
  as secondary respiratory muscle, 26
Scholten, Dr. Jeffrey, 3
Seated postures with ball
  Bridge to Modified Bow, 70
  Eagle pose, 69
  sitting on ball, 68
  Warrior II pose, 71

Secondary respiratory muscles, 26–27, 39
  emotional response from breathing with, 27
Semimembranosus, 22
Semitendinosus, 22
Serratus anterior, 21, 24
Shallow breathing, 28
Sheng-yen, 45
Shoulder and neck tension, due to weak inner core, 25
Shoulder girdle
  stabilizing with Downward Facing Dog, 66–67
  stabilizing with Handstand, 66–67
  stabilizing with Plank pose, 55, 66
  stabilizing with Upward Facing Dog, 65
Shoulders, cultivating pure movement at, 11
Side Plank, 57, 91. See also Plank pose
  on BOSU Balance Trainer
    as strength- and stability-challenging pose, 89
    as strength-enhancing activation pose, 88
    variation 1, 77
      increasing speed to flutter, 77
    variation 2, 77
    variation 3, 77
  as strength-enhancing activation pose, 88
Sitting on ball, 68
  as activation pose, 87
Skeletal muscles, postural and phasic functions, 18–19
Sockman, Ralph W., 58
Soleus, 22
Specific Adaptations to Imposed Demands (SAID), 46
Speed of movement, increasing for stability challenge, 47
Spinal flexion, exhalation during, 28
Spine
  as central axis, 11
  as core, 11
  inner core and stability of, 25
Stability ball
  balance challenges using, 60
  ball to belly postures, 65–67
  base of support using, 60
  Bridge to Modified Bow poses with, 70
  Cat pose with, 63
  core strengthening with, 59–60
  Downward Facing Dog with, 66–67
  Eagle pose on, 69
  figure four hip opener with, 62
  Handstand with, 66–67
  kneeling postures with, 63–64
  Kneeling Tadasana on, 64
  Little Bridge pose with, 62

Index

About Functional Synergy

Functional Synergy was founded in 1999 by Susi Hately Aldous. It is the first known yoga studio in North America offering customized yoga programs for people with injury, illness, or really tight bodies.

Functional Synergy remains innovative while teaching people how to find quiet, how to rest, and how to cultivate ease, strength, and stabilization both "on the mat" and "off the mat," whether they are elite athletes, weekend warriors, desk jockeys, or parents racing after children.

If you would like more information on Functional Synergy and its programs for people with pain or injury, please call **403.229.2617**, toll free at **1.866.229.2645**, or visit **www.functionalsynergy.com.**

Deepen Your Practice
Online Education

Going Deeper: Learning More Anatomy

If you loved this book and want to learn more about anatomy as it relates to yoga, your core stability, and other aspects of yoga asana, our free monthly ezine, I Love Anatomy, is for you.

To receive our free monthly ezine, please visit
www.anatomyandasana.com.

(Like you, we don't like SPAM. We won't in any way sell, trade, or share your email address. It is used to send you our free ezine and provide you with updates on upcoming courses and workshops.)

About Functional Synergy

Functional Synergy was founded in 1999 by Susi Hately Aldous. It is the first known yoga studio in North America offering customized yoga programs for people with injury, illness, or really tight bodies.

Functional Synergy remains innovative while teaching people how to find quiet, how to rest, and how to cultivate ease, strength, and stabilization both "on the mat" and "off the mat," whether they are elite athletes, weekend warriors, desk jockeys, or parents racing after children.

If you would like more information on Functional Synergy and its programs for people with pain or injury, please call **403.229.2617**, toll free at **1.866.229.2645**, or visit **www.functionalsynergy.com**.

Deepen Your Practice
Online Education

Going Deeper: Learning More Anatomy

If you loved this book and want to learn more
about anatomy as it relates to yoga, your core stability,
and other aspects of yoga asana, our free monthly
ezine, I Love Anatomy, is for you.

To receive our free monthly ezine, please visit
www.anatomyandasana.com.

*(Like you, we don't like SPAM. We won't in any way
sell, trade, or share your email address. It is used to send
you our free ezine and provide you with updates on
upcoming courses and workshops.)*